Stroke at a

at a
Stroke

The rollercoaster of living with someone who has had a stroke

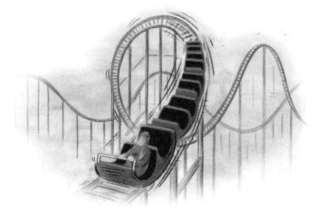

Huw Watkins

Editors Richard Craze, Roni Jay

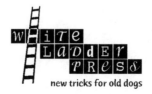

new tricks for old dogs

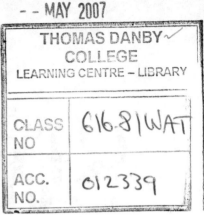
Published by White Ladder Press Ltd
Great Ambrook, Near Ipplepen, Devon TQ12 5UL
01803 813343
www.whiteladderpress.com

First published in Great Britain in 2006

10 9 8 7 6 5 4 3 2 1

© Huw Watkins 2006

The right of Huw Watkins to be identified as author of this work has been asserted by him in accordance with the Copyright, Designs and Patents Act 1988.

ISBN 0 9548219 9 8
ISBN 978 0 9548219 9 9

British Library Cataloguing in Publication Data
A CIP record for this book can be obtained from the British Library.

Designed and typeset by Julie Martin Ltd
Cover design by Julie Martin Ltd
Cover illustration by Chris Mutter
Cover printed by St Austell Printing Company
Printed and bound by TJ International Ltd, Padstow, Cornwall

White Ladder Press
Great Ambrook, Near Ipplepen, Devon TQ12 5UL
01803 813343
www.whiteladderpress.com

Names and places in this narrative have been changed: the events in the narrative occurred as described.

All author royalties from the sale of this book will be donated to Different Strokes.

Acknowledgements and thanks

The need to write this account sprang from the very direct experience of coping with the devastating impact that a stroke can have on the lives of many people. So my first thanks go to the various members of the Health Services who appear in these pages, and who gave so much help in so many different ways. The relatives and friends who offered such magnificent support are too numerous to list, but if you recognise yourself in the narrative, thanks again.

Four friends read the typescript and provided detailed and insightful comments. So thank you JB, DG, RH and DW. Your reactions were most helpful.

Although the suggestions in the book are based on practical experience, this has been backed up by information obtained from various voluntary organisations, and I appreciate that too.

LH was willing to talk openly with me about his own feelings and reactions on suffering a stroke, as did Mike Ripley, whose own book 'Surviving a Stroke', covers this personal experience comprehensively. My particular thanks go to my editors, Roni Jay and Richard Craze, who guided the book through its various drafts, and acted as a conduit for comments from their board. Their very helpful and constructive suggestions have been the major influence on shaping the structure of the book.

Lastly, but most importantly, I pay tribute to the two stroke patients, to Bob, whose recovery was an inspiration to everyone, and to Dilys, the central character, whose courage can only be imagined, and in whose memory this book has been written.

HW

Prologue

The third biggest cause of death, and the major cause of serious disability in the UK, is a stroke. Various books describe the experiences of the victim of a stroke, but little has been written to help the relatives. Some are young, but many are elderly, shocked, trying to come to terms with uncertain and possibly fatal damage to a loved one, and often to major changes in their own lives.

This book is written from the diary I kept at the time of my late wife's stroke. It is essentially a story of a couple's journey across a summer, and the narrative covers the many shocks and uncertainties encountered along the way. The information panels in the book offer practical suggestions for helping with these difficulties, many of which apply to someone coping with a partner's serious illness, whether from a stroke or otherwise. In addition, a short list of some useful sources of information appears on the publisher's website, **www.whiteladderpress.com**. Readers without access to the internet can obtain a free copy by phoning or writing to White Ladder (see contact details on page 166).

For one partner, the summer's journey led from life to death; for the other, it led from an old life to a new one. It is the latter journey, a voyage from despair to hope, on which the book concentrates.

HW

June 23rd afternoon

I was at home when the phone rang: it was the GP.

"I've just heard from the senior registrar at St. Michael's," she said. "They've made a diagnosis, and Dilys has had a brain-stem stroke. I really can't tell you any more," the GP went on, anticipating my questions. "You need to see Dr. Phillips, the consultant to the hospital. He's an excellent fellow, very approachable and very well thought of." And the GP rang off.

What's a brainstem stroke, I wondered.

John, our older son, was visiting Dilys that afternoon. By chance, it was a day when Dr. Phillips happened to be con-sulting at St. Michael's, and John had managed to have a word with him.

"He's very clear and direct," John said when I saw him later, obviously impressed. "He told me he was certain that Mum has had a brainstem stroke. But I'm afraid he also said that the future was very uncertain."

I tried to absorb these two pieces of news: a brainstem stroke and a very uncertain future.

"He wants to send Mum over to the main hospital for a brain-stem scan," John went on. "Apparently it's a different proce-dure from the ordinary scan. He wants to know whether there's bleeding going on."

Bleeding: I tried to absorb this, too.

"I brought these leaflets from the hospital. They might be helpful," John said.

I took John to his train. When I got back home, I glanced at the leaflets he had brought, picking out a phrase that was aimed at the relatives of stroke patients.

"You'll find you'll be riding an emotional rollercoaster," it said.

How true that phrase proved for me, and doubtless for many others who have watched their loved ones trying to recover from an illness that might have devastating results – but might not. Where the victim is in hospital, and all the care is in the hands of others, there is little the relatives can do, except watch, wear the mask of encouragement, hope for maximum recovery and prepare for what might be very changed circumstances. Every relative of a stroke victim must be ready to live the hopes and fears of an uncertain future.

I cast my mind back over the preceding five weeks.

Third week of May

Dilys wanted a new pair of sandals for the summer to come, so we were walking down the long High Street towards the shoe shops. The spring morning was bright with the promise of a sunny day. How did our local population manage to support so many shoe shops, I wondered idly, seeing the racks of special offers claiming attention on the pavements ahead. Should be time for a quick coffee after the sandals, and then home for lunch.

We were both retired, sharing the sunshine with so many others. I'll spend the afternoon gardening, preparing the ground for planting beans, I thought. Thursday: so we had the bridge club that evening. Looked like another enjoyable retirement day.

"Huw, I don't feel very well."

Dilys stopped suddenly, and put her hand on my arm. People flowed past us, intent on their own purposes, chatting, smiling, while we alone stood still.

May 15th, nearly 11 o'clock.

"What's the matter?"

"I think I might have had a little stroke. Can you take me back to the car?"

We returned to the car park, her arm in mine. No one took any notice of the brown haired lady, dressed in blouse and skirt,

her usually smiling face now pale and set. She had no problems in walking, though she was walking rather slowly, I
noticed. "What's the feeling?" I asked. She shook her head.

"Just want to get home." She clearly didn't want to talk.

My mind jumped back to a couple of years ago. After complaining of "feeling distant; not with it" on two or three occasions, Dilys had been seen by a consultant, who had diagnosed
a series of TIAs (see below), or minor strokes, and prescribed
a daily aspirin. Before then, strokes were events that happened to other people, and our reaction was a mixture of ignorance and anxiety. So I'd got hold of a booklet from the Stroke
Association, and we'd learnt more about TIAs. We learnt how
they're caused, we'd been reassured by the discussion on
treatment, and then gradually we let everything fade to the
back of our minds as life continued normally. Two years without a recurrence: you feel the danger has gone away for good.

Most people have heard the term 'stroke' and to many it conjures up the
mixed feelings of ignorance and anxiety mentioned above. TIAs (standing for transient ischaemic attacks) are actually minor strokes, or minor
injuries to the brain. There are two sorts. In one the blood supply to the
brain is reduced, perhaps by a clot, or by narrowing or kinking of an
artery. In the other, a blood vessel in the brain actually bursts. In both
cases brain cells die.

The unwell feeling usually goes after a few hours, but in spite of feeling
better it is important that your relative or partner sees a doctor as soon
as possible. Once the feeling of illness disappears, people can be reluc-

tant to trouble busy doctors. Persuade them otherwise: early investigation and treatment can help to prevent a more serious stroke occurring.

A stroke is a major TIA, in which the symptoms persist. Details of TIAs and other information about the different kinds of strokes can be found in the very useful pamphlets of the Stroke Association (contact details on the White Ladder website). The pamphlets cover many issues, including medication, rehabilitation and a preventive surgical procedure (carotid endarterectomy) which can sometimes be used to widen arteries whose constriction threatens to lead to a serious stroke.

Back home, she went to bed. This was the pattern of the previous sequence of TIAs, straight to bed, sleep soundly for a couple of hours, and then get up quietly. I felt worried. Were the TIAs returning, in spite of the aspirin, and if so, what treatment would be prescribed? But Dilys didn't get up. She slept most of the rest of the day, bedroom curtains drawn, waking occasionally when I suggested something to eat. But she didn't want to eat. Even her favourite light sandwich was refused.

"The food tastes funny," she said.

This was not the stroke, I thought; the pattern's different. What's wrong?

Over the last couple of months Dilys had been to see the GP three times, complaining of giddiness and feeling unwell, an unspecified feeling, the sort of amorphous problem that gives no clues. Tablets for giddiness had had no effect, and no cause had been found.

The GP had turned to me on the last visit and asked, "Do you think Dilys is depressed?"

I recalled that Dilys had had a short period of severe depression 20 years ago, and this must be in her medical notes. I thought carefully. The doctor was exploring possibilities, and truth was important. I looked straight at Dilys and smiled at her.

"She would be the first to acknowledge that she's not always one of life's optimists," I said. Dilys grinned wryly back, and I felt pleased at her reaction. "But I know when she's depressed, and she's not depressed now. She's worried and unhappy about feeling ill, but she's not depressed."

Dilys was a very practical person. She usually looked carefully at a situation, not willing to take a risk until she'd satisfied herself that there weren't hidden problems. Her judgement was excellent, and she'd have made an excellent businesswoman, though in fact, she made an excellent teacher. We'd met during our year of teacher training in London, she intending to teach languages, and I science. Our courses were therefore different, and we didn't see each other in the week. What brought us together was an October youth hostel weekend when, on the train down to Sussex, I sat opposite this attractive, brown haired, brown eyed 21 year old, and offered to lend her my map.

"Where exactly are we going?" she asked, looking uncertainly at the sheet. So of course I moved across to show her.

In those early post-war days, universities and colleges were swamped by applications from men and women returning from the forces and from national service. To try to compensate these servicemen for the time they'd given to the country, they were often allowed to enter courses as soon as they were 'demobbed', i.e. freed from national service, rather than having to wait until the usual September start. Dilys had come straight from her degree, starting in September as normal, whereas I had entered the previous January, and so in a couple of months my year would have finished, and I'd be off teaching. Just two months to get to know her. Time was short!

In those days, student hostels weren't mixed, but we did eat together, and the weekly 'hop' or dance gave more opportunities for meeting. By December, we were seeing each other regularly, and in January I'd taken a job in the London area.

The following year we married. More than 50 years later, we still teased each other about that map.

She'd been a wonderful wife, supporting me loyally when I returned to full time study, bringing up our three children, and sacrificing her own career to foster mine. She'd been brought up in a family where her parents had had to struggle to make ends meet, and I'd learnt a lot about the virtues of thrift and hard work from her. But she wasn't a one sided character. She possessed that essential trait of a good teacher – a real sense of humour, which bubbled up in the family as well as in the classroom, and her repartee was second to none. In the marriage lottery, I'd been very lucky.

"Best day's work I ever did," I always said whenever she needed to talk about it.

No, she wasn't depressed.

Back home, after the abortive shoe shopping expedition, and still in bed, she complained of pain. "My teeth hurt," she said. "And my eye," she pointed to her right eye, "and neck. All down this side of my head.

"I must see the dentist. There's something very wrong with my teeth." Dilys was very proud of her almost perfect teeth, so I wasn't surprised that she was worried about them. Yet it was strange: she'd had a dental check-up just a few weeks ago. I rang the dentist and arranged an emergency appointment for the next day.

She slept all night. The next morning she wasn't feeling well enough to travel the 12 miles to the dental surgery. I cancelled the appointment.

At lunchtime she took a little mushroom soup, and half a tomato sandwich. Starting to eat! I felt the first ripple of relief, even though Dilys herself was still in some pain. We'd tried painkillers, but with no apparent effect.

"I'll ring the doctor," I said.

She refused. "No, don't. I've bothered her enough recently. Leave it for the time being."

Now Dilys was a strong character, who always knew her own mind. She liked the GP, and there was no antipathy there. I offered again, but she was adamant. After more than 50 years together, I knew what she was thinking.

"I'll see her when I'm well enough to go to the surgery. I've got a follow-up appointment for Wednesday, so I'll see her then."

Exactly what I thought. She hated bothering people – always had. Pity she was so determined. I felt uneasy about her decision. But at least she was positive, expecting to get better. So I felt a little better myself.

All strokes are different, and it's easy for patients and relatives (and sometimes doctors) to be misled by different symptoms from those encountered previously. It is sometimes easy to go down the wrong route. If you think that the problems might be related to a previous stroke, don't hesitate to raise your query with the doctor: patients sometimes have the best, instinctive feeling about their illness, and if they're wrong there's no harm in having asked the question, and considerable benefit in being reassured. The principle is to get specialist advice as soon as possible. Again, it's particularly important for relatives to insist on this.

It was now the weekend. As usual the three children rang. Like all parents, we always call them the 'children', even though they're all married, and have produced some super grandchildren.

"Mum's just not quite herself," I lied, when she didn't come to the phone. "Nothing serious, just having a rest in bed."

Neither of us wanted to worry them unnecessarily. After all, she would be her old self again in a day or two, wouldn't she? But there were no signs of it yet, and a question now began to appear, rather like an evil genius peeping out of the theatre wings: was this something more, something different, something that might be a serious illness?

Dilys stayed in bed, curtains shut. She still was hardly eating, just a little mushroom soup at lunchtime. I offered breakfast, tea, supper. "No thanks, I just don't want it." Now her chief worry was her right eye: "It's funny; I can't see properly out of it." And the teeth and mouth generally didn't feel right. "The right side of my face aches," she said. She had no temperature, and still didn't want to bother the doctor.

When the weekend was over, she tried to get up.

Dilys loved to sit in 'her' chair by the lounge window, enjoying the fine view over the valley to the mountains beyond. The white farmhouses sat below small fields that led up to the open grazing of the mountainsides above. That day, she walked to the window in her dressing gown, but I noticed that she needed my arm, and her walk was tentative and slow, obviously an effort for her. I sat her down in the chair. But after 10 minutes she asked to be taken back to bed.

"I feel so tired," she said. This wasn't Dilys at all. The active, sociable girl, with the ready wit and quick riposte had gone. Although she was still expecting to get to the Health Centre for the Wednesday appointment with the doctor, I was beginning to have doubts.

On Tuesday, a new problem: she was worried that her bowels weren't operating.

"Don't worry," I reassured. "You've eaten hardly anything. You've nothing to go on."

"But it doesn't feel right," she said.

When the patient isn't eating it's too easy for the carer, now eating alone, not to bother much about meals. You need to eat well yourself. If your cooking isn't up to much, order a meal from a take-away, or ask a neighbour to buy you some ready meals.

She clearly was in no position to travel to the Health Centre tomorrow. I told her I'd use her appointment to see the doctor myself, and explain her problems. She didn't object: she had now been unwell for five days, and I was worried.

Her doctor appeared at the door of the waiting room, and called her name. Dr. Jean Stewart was a young, well liked GP, probably in her late twenties, round faced, short fair hair, and blue eyes behind a pair of metal framed glasses. She had one of those warm smiles that immediately puts people at ease. I entered the consulting room, and explained that I was here to discuss Dilys's problems.

"Does she know you're here?" the pleasant GP asked. I was slightly surprised that she thought I might have come to talk about Dilys without her knowledge. But it was a sensible question, I realised afterwards.

I described her symptoms; the lack of appetite, the sleeping, the facial and dental pain, the loss of independent walking. As I did so, something happened that hadn't happened to me since I was a child. I started to cry. And I couldn't stop. For fully several minutes I sat there weeping while the GP told me that it was quite all right to cry, and waited for me to finish. Oh God, what shame, crying for no apparent reason. I hadn't even cried when my parents died. At last I was able to put the handkerchief away.

"I'll call to see her," she said, "but I'm away tomorrow, so it'll be Friday."

Stress is only to be expected when a relative is ill, and often relatives sense the seriousness of a situation more deeply than the patient or the doctor. The relative knows the patient so well, and is aware how uncharacteristic are the differences in behaviour and reactions that the patient shows. And when the cause of the problem and its possible outcome are not known, this adds to the stress. It is the start of the emotional rollercoaster.

I felt a great relief. Someone was coming to do something. And the relief was mixed with a little shame that I should have been unable to describe Dilys's illness – for illness is what it had now become – without breaking down in such an unmanly fashion. Why did you break down like that, I wondered to myself. It's Dilys who's ill, not you. Had the last few days really been so stressful, so much more stressful than I had appreciated? We'd been through so much in our life together – our babies unwell, our parents' deaths, our own illnesses – without crumpling like that. Why did this have such an effect? Was it because I was carrying the worry alone, hiding my concern from her and the family?

It's natural to want to protect the children from unnecessary worry, particularly if the likely outcome is positive, and the children are young. But if not, bring them into the picture: they need to know and can be the best support. Even young children, who are likely to be living at home and to be aware of the illness, need honest information given in a non-threatening way. Use your judgement.

I walked red eyed through the waiting room, looking straight ahead so as not to have to acknowledge anyone, and hoping that no one I knew would spot my condition.

When I got home I told Dilys that the doctor would be calling. She didn't seem unduly pleased, and didn't complain about having to wait till Friday. Secretly I wished with all my heart that I had disregarded her wishes, and been in touch with the doctor before, for my sake as much as hers. But it was now tremendously reassuring to know that the Health Service was bringing support.

Once again, see the doctor as soon as possible. It's easy to be too aware of advice not to overburden the GP. If you're really worried, your doctor will be happy either to reassure you or else they'll be able to take action early, always important in any illness.

And don't hesitate to override your partner's reluctance to bother the

GP. If it turns out to be a false alarm, and the hesitation was justified, so what? The risk of it being something serious is not worth taking. Think of yourself, as well as your partner; you want to do the best for him or her, and anything less is demeaning to both of you.

Once again, share your worries with the family. You may think it's brave to hide them, and right not to bother others, and just occasionally that may be right. But think how you'd feel if your parent/sibling were ill and you weren't told, because someone felt the need to protect you. A key concept is trust. The family must be able to feel that you can be trusted to tell the truth and not conceal it. So your worries should be brought out in the open; others' views are often helpful, and can lend support to any action you are thinking of taking.

That afternoon I dashed into town for some food shopping. As I passed the shoe shops where Dilys had hoped to buy her sandals for the summer, I wondered how soon it would be before we'd get them.

Fourth week of May

The GP's car drew up outside. I felt a great sense of relief; someone seeing Dilys at last. The GP sat on the side of the bed, as pleasant and as cheerful as ever, putting Dilys at ease at once, chatting away about the weather and telling Dilys about her children. Blood pressure, temperature – both fine, she found. It was the teeth and mouth problem that exercised her most, and after a careful examination, she diagnosed a case of thrush, and prescribed antibiotics and a mouthwash. For the constipation, which was worrying Dilys, she arranged for the nurse to call and administer an enema.

"Come and see me on Tuesday," the GP said to Dilys. I felt a weight lifting off my shoulders. The doctor was clearly expecting a rapid improvement.

I hurried to the chemist, and we started the treatment at once.

The nurse came the following day, a lively, talkative lady, who soon dispelled any embarrassment Dilys felt over the enema. It was the day that would have been the start of our family holiday in Majorca, a holiday I'd had to cancel a few weeks ago, when Dilys had started to feel unwell. The nurse was encouraging.

"You were wise to cancel," she said. "It's a lovely island, and you'll enjoy it so much more when you're both fit."

The company seemed to be doing Dilys good. For the moment, her old self peeped out from behind the curtain of her illness, a glimpse of the lively, sociable, clear voiced person I knew so well.

To cheer Dilys up I began to talk about where she'd like to go when she was better.

"Somewhere in this country at first," she thought. "The Lakes – I've always liked the Lakes." I talked about some of our various holidays there, renting cottages in Coniston and Dunnerdale, staying in Langdale, and our last trip there, a jolly weekend with a lot of friends near Ambleside.

"Definitely the Lakes," she said. Then the nurse left, and she fell back to sleep.

The weekend passed without any obvious change in the feeling in Dilys's throat.

"It takes a couple of days for the antibiotic to work," I encouraged her.

The boys and their families had now arrived in Majorca, where we would all have been on holiday together, and they rang us.

"Much the same," I answered. "Still resting in bed, but the doctor's been and she's on tablets now."

"And how about you?" they asked.

"Oh I'm fine." They sounded reassured.

Calls from the children really help. Knowing that someone else is concerned about the invalid eases the pressure of your concern: others share it with you. And it's a good feeling to know that they're thinking of you, too.

On Monday, for the first time, she wanted an arm to walk the five steps to the toilet. "I'm feeling very wobbly," she said, "and I don't want to fall." Our bedroom has an en suite bathroom, and the toilet is five paces from the bed. Yet when she went to urinate, she now needed my arm for those five paces. Why is her walking deteriorating, I wondered. Is it just weakness, or something more?

I felt a sudden hollow, helpless feeling. The relief at the doctor's optimism dwindled and the worry I had felt last week reappeared, joined by a sense of foreboding. Still hardly eating, and now the walking beginning to go? Later in the day, after half a bowl of soup for lunch, she thought she'd get up again, and sit in her favourite window seat. She took my arm again, and we started for the lounge. I noticed how slowly she was walking, and when we got to the hall, a few yards away, she asked to sit down. "I need a little rest," she said. After a minute or two she started again, and we reached the lounge.

It was a beautiful day; across the valley the sun shone on the hills to the south, and the flowers she loved in the garden were sitting up as if in salute. "It's no good," she said after 10 minutes, "I've got to get back to bed." She slept for the rest of the day. It was if she'd had an energetic workout: but she'd just walked 20 yards, with great difficulty. I cancelled a day trip we had booked for the following week.

If you're worried about calling the doctor yet again, don't forget the NHS Direct helpline. There's always a trained person there to talk things through with you. The phone number is in the Helpline page at the front of the telephone directory.

"Washing day," Dilys reminded me.

"Put in the powder and press the button?" I asked uncertainly. At least I knew where the machine was, and it ought to be foolproof.

She nodded. "No need to change the programme."

Thank the Lord for that, I thought. I had done the washing occasionally in the past, and now wasn't the time to have to learn the intricacies of the household gadgets. I was a member of that older generation where household tasks were strictly the responsibility of the females, and apart from a long ago year at university, I'd not looked after myself. I felt that camping trips in the wild had made me pretty self-sufficient, but washing clothes in a stream and cooking over a primus stove wasn't the best of training for running a household with an invalid.

There was no change the next morning, except that the pain in her eye was worse. I rang the medical centre and waited till the end of the morning, when the doctor rang back.

"I'll arrange an appointment this afternoon for the eye clinic," she said. She explained about the need to check for arteritis, a possible complication of the polymyalgia from which Dilys had been steadily recovering.

"But I can't get her there without an ambulance."

I described her difficulties in getting to the lounge. Trying to dress her, getting her to the car, walking from the hospital car park into the main building.....impossible. The doctor thought for a moment.

"We'll check via a blood test," she said. "I'll get the nurse to call in this afternoon to take a sample, and if you can get the sample to the path. lab I'll ask for an urgent test. They'll phone me with the results and I'll let you know tomorrow."

The nurse came that afternoon. Before I drove off to catch the hospital pathology lab with the blood sample, nurse asked if I would like her to arrange a wheelchair for Dilys.

Dilys in a wheelchair? After all these years of health, had poor Dilys suddenly come to this? It was another blow: but of course it made sense. I agreed to fetch the chair from a centre some 20 miles away the next morning, and drove off for the path. lab.

Next day everything seemed to happen. I left Dilys, who still wasn't eating breakfast, found the wheelchair centre without too much difficulty and returned to her. When I got back, we tried to chat for a while, and, oh dear, I noticed a slight slurring in her speech. Yet another blow. What was going on, I wondered. Later, she asked for help to get to the toilet, but she wasn't able to get there in time. The dreaded word 'incontinence' flashed through my mind. Was this just a one-off, or the shape of things to come? Foreboding grew. Then the doctor rang.

"The tests are completely clear," she said. Perhaps I should have been glad that the possible arteritis had been excluded; in fact I was much more worried that the cause of Dilys's illness had not been identified. I couldn't wait to describe the latest symptoms to the doctor. There was a distinct pause.

Most people think of a serious stroke as a sudden, devastating loss of functions. This is often the case, but not always. When someone has already suffered from TIAs, or is known to be vulnerable to a stroke, that possibility must always be considered. Those of us who are not medics are unlikely to be aware of the range of symptoms which might indicate a stroke and to be able to distinguish them from other possibilities.

"I'll call to see her tomorrow," she said.

True to her word, the GP arrived in the morning. When I opened the door to her, she stopped in the hall before going into the bedroom.

"I'm beginning to be concerned about Dilys," she warned. My sense of foreboding became overwhelming, and I rapidly rattled off my worries.

"So many of her functions – walking, speech, bladder control, all these now seem to be deteriorating," I stated anxiously, "as well as the original problems, the loss of appetite and pain round the side of her head and eye."

"Sometimes minor problems can mask something more serious," she continued, "and I might have to suggest admission to hospital. How would you feel about that?"

I felt a sense of relief that something more was being done, and said so.

"Then let's talk to Dilys together," she said.

Dilys was reluctant. I could guess what she was thinking....she'd seen others leaving the security and comfort of their homes for hospital investigations whose outcomes were always uncertain. The GP and I tried to persuade her.

"You've been in hospital before," I reminded her. She nodded, unhappily.

"And the treatment facilities are so much better than we can provide at home," the GP supported.

"Will you promise I'll come back here?" Dilys asked.

"Of course," I promised. "Once they've found out what's wrong, and got you well again, of course you'll come home. I promise."

It's important to be very careful over promises. It's too easy to promise what you can't fulfil, even if you put in a condition. In this case the condition was "once you're well again," so in one sense the promise was fair. But it would have been fairer if I'd said something like "No one can ever promise that, Dilys, but I will promise that once you're well again......"

Doctors are far more familiar with symptoms than the laity. But you yourself are more familiar with your partner than the doctor – which is why the GP very sensibly had earlier asked me about Dilys and depression. Sometimes you can sense the severity of changes in your partner's condition more easily than the doctor, and if you feel that, it's right to say so. In this situation I just felt from my very first visit to the doctor that something was really wrong, even though I couldn't identify it. If you feel that, be ready to say so, strongly.

Dilys trusted me, I knew that. And so I gave a promise that I hoped and thought would be honoured, though in my heart I knew it just might not be. The promise persuaded her. The GP rang the hospital and arranged for an ambulance to call that afternoon.

First week of June

It was the day after I'd accompanied Dilys into the large district hospital. I wondered at the ease with which two cheerful ambulance men had lifted her on to a stretcher, and then realised that she must have lost some weight; it was just over a fortnight since she'd eaten anything substantial. I drove after the ambulance, and followed her into the emergency admissions ward. The admissions nurse seemed rather remote, bored with what to her must have been a dull routine of thermometers and tourniquets, the usual measurements of temperature and blood pressure.

Dilys seemed quiet when I visited, though very glad to see me. I kissed her, and started to look for a vase for the flowers I'd brought.

"I fell last night," she said at once, interrupting my search. "I was trying to get to the loo, and I fell. I've been down for an x-ray."

I put the flowers down. She'd been allowed to fall! I felt very angry: a fortnight at home and there hadn't been a problem, 12 hours in hospital and this happens. "Did you ring for a nurse?" I asked.

She nodded. "No one came. But I'll be moved today to another ward."

We chatted for a while, and then I went off to find out what had happened. Sister was quite direct. "Yes, she tried to get to the toilet in the night, but she fell in the ward, hitting her head. We arranged for a skull x-ray, and everything is all right."

"She tells me she rang for help," I said.

"The night staff were very busy last night," Sister said, "and I can understand that they might not have been able to come at once."

I said nothing; a complaint against overworked staff would be inappropriate.

A patient is someone who shows patience. It's always better to ask for information before complaining about treatment. Hospital staff are busy, often overworked, and like any one of us, don't take kindly to ill-founded criticism.

At the same time, a patient is in a weak position, needing someone to act as an advocate, so have no hesitation in raising questions if he or she – or you – is unhappy.

On my second visit that day Dilys had indeed been moved into another ward. She would be in the care of Dr. Feldman, a consultant she'd seen a couple of years ago, when her TIAs had been diagnosed. It was a weekend, and no investigations would start for a couple of days.

Her bed was at the end of the ward. From it, Dilys could see a beautiful view of green hillsides sweeping up to moorland. That early June enjoyed a spell of wonderful sunshine, white fine weather clouds sailed across the skyline, and Dilys liked watching the shadows marching over the mountains. Cards had already started to arrive, and the first friends called that evening. The news was getting round.

"I hear she's not eating," one said to me at the door. I nodded.

"She should be getting high energy drinks," the friend said. "You ask for them, if she's not getting them."

What were these high energy drinks? I wondered. Lucozade or something? On her table was a full carafe of water. The level didn't seem to change, and she never wanted more than a sip when I tried to help. Would these high energy things help? I went to Staff Nurse, sitting in the ward office, writing away, and asked.

"We'll bring some," she said, and shortly afterwards a nurse came by with two packets of drink. When I opened one for her, Dilys wrinkled up her nose. "Don't want it," she said.

By the bed was a state-of-the-art media unit, telephone, tv and radio with earphones. It wasn't being used.

"Can you get Radio 4 for me?" she asked. "I can't manage this thing."

Dilys is not very technically minded, but she has no difficulty with home media equipment, even mastering the supreme test, the video recorder, with ease. So I was a little surprised at her request.

"I'm tired," she said. I left her with Radio 4 playing through the earphones.

Entertainment can be helpful, but not if it needs too much attention. Patients are often tired, and something undemanding, like soothing music, may be better than a quiz show. Radio, to which eyes can be closed, is often a better medium than television while patients are still feeling weary.

If the hospital doesn't have easily managed facilities, think of bringing in a portable radio, but remember the earphones: not everyone wants to hear someone else's favourite programme.

Monday came. Many visitors were arriving now, bringing little gifts of flowers, which she appreciated, and chocolate, which she couldn't eat. I asked them not to stay too long; I knew how tired Dilys now felt.

At the risk of overkill, it's worth repeating how tired patients, perhaps especially stroke patients, often feel, and how important it is for visitors, however well meaning, to be restricted until the patient is ready. There is a time in recovery from a stroke when stimulation is more important than rest, and that's something over which the hospital staff can advise. Then, cheerful, understanding visitors, talking about familiar events, are welcome indeed. Until then, it may be better to keep visiting to close family only.

For me, a routine was now being established: household chores and shopping in the morning, then lunch and straight to the hospital for the first visiting period. There was time to get home for an early evening meal, and then back for the second visiting period.

Our daughter in New Zealand rang me.

"I'm holding a flight in case I ought to come over," she said. I was shaken for a moment. Flying over! Janet must think this is serious to consider leaving her young children.

"No need to, really not," I said. "Mum's not well, but she's being looked after in hospital. I'll certainly let you know if you need to come over."

"How are you managing?" she asked.

"Fine," I replied. Washing had become a routine, and cooking for one was easy.

Women on their own don't usually need advice on running a household, but for men, especially older men, routine is the key. Make a washing plan which, apart from the weekly clothes, gives a regular turn to those other things like sheets, pillowcases, towels (bathroom and kitchen) bathroom mats, duvet covers etc, and stick to the plan.

Remember short cuts. If you sleep in a double bed there's no need to wash the sheets as often as when two of you use them: rotate them through 180 and use them again before washing.

If you're cooking, use the freezer; don't just cook for one, but cook enough for four or six. Divide into portions, freeze separately and you'll have your own ready meals in the freezer.

Remember to read labels carefully before buying food: not all food freezes. I like crème caramels, bought 10 of them, only to find that they don't freeze. I had to eat them all in the next few days. (But I enjoyed it.)

And don't feel too proud to ask for advice.

At this stage of the illness, I was learning the basics of running a household. I wasn't worried about cleaning – the house doesn't get too dirty with just one in it, I told myself, and the occasional hoover over the carpets and the occasional clean of the kitchen floor seemed to be enough. More proficiency came later.

Janet told me she'd phoned to Dilys's bedside, but Dilys hadn't been able to take the call. What a shame, I thought. I knew how pleased Dilys would be to talk to her. And it was yet another little sign of deterioration, another little blow to my hopes for her.

"Ring when I'm there," I arranged with Janet. She did, and I gave the phone to Dilys, whose face lit up with pleasure.

For someone suddenly finding themselves in the strange surroundings of a hospital ward, contact with family, even at the earliest stages of a stroke, is reassuring and helpful. A personal visit is better than ringing in to the bedside, but a phone call from far away family members, perhaps particularly children, can still be a wonderful encouragement. Ringing home to find how the patient is doing is important, but don't forget about a brief call direct to the patient.

Contact from friends is a different matter. A stream of telephone calls to the house, however well meaning, can be irritating. And they so often come when the meal is ready to eat, or you're ready to sit and relax after a busy day. For friends, cards are a much more convenient way of showing interest and support.

On Tuesday the consultant did his ward round. At last, I thought. Now we'll hear what he thinks the problem is, and what to do about it. I went straight to Dilys's bedside as soon as the ward round was over and visitors were allowed in.

"I'm to have a brain scan," she said. At last, I thought; something being done. My heart lifted. "Good," I smiled, trying to encourage her. "Now we'll get somewhere."

Dilys's favourite fruits are cherries. The first Kent cherries had arrived in the shops and I brought some in for her. If she'd eat anything, she'd eat those. She managed to eat a couple, very slowly I noticed, but then nearly choked and stopped.

"It's no good," she said sadly, "I can't eat them."

I felt that hollow, empty feeling again. Yesterday, the news of the scan to come had cheered me; today, her obvious misery at her own inabilities depressed me.

I encouraged her to take a sip of water from her carafe. I tried to help her with her meals, with very little success. These were delivered on trays by the catering staff, who took them away uneaten, making no comment. Catering seemed to be an arrangement independent of the nurses, who appeared to have little or no interest in Dilys's eating and drinking. I had to see the consultant, I felt, on several counts. She really hadn't eaten for a fortnight. Did he know this, I wondered. I saw Sister, who seemed surprised that I wanted to see him.

"Try to catch him after his ward round tomorrow," she said.

I hung around the ward until at last the consultant emerged, heading for the exit. I ran up to catch him before he disappeared.

"Dilys Watkins...." He stopped in his tracks, and pondered for a second. Someone so important to me, just one among so many to him, I thought.

"Ah yes," he said. "The good news is that the blood tests are all fine, and we're waiting for the scan results. Don't worry, we'll get to the bottom of this," and with an encouraging smile he turned, and continued his dash for the exit before I could ask another question.

The following day, a drip had been inserted: she was getting fluids at last. I felt relieved.

Dilys had her brain scan on Thursday.

"The scan was all clear," she said when I came to see her. I felt more relief; several nasty possibilities had been ruled out. "Good," I encouraged.

As usual, she was sitting up in a chair, looking pale and drawn.

"Now get me back to bed, Huw," she pleaded.

The nurses insisted that she sat in the chair – standard practice to avoid bedsores, I assumed. But I couldn't resist her request, whatever the nurses thought, and her relief as I helped her up on to the bed was obvious.

A new lady arrived and introduced herself.

"I'm the physiotherapist. I'm here to help Dilys with her walking.

Good, I thought; more support.

There is a team of different professionals whose skills are used to help stroke victims. Physiotherapists work with stroke patients (and others) who have problems over mobility and balance. They see their patients both while they're in hospital and, if resources permit, after the return home. It's often valuable for relatives to be present when the physio helps the patient. It's an opportunity to learn from the professional the right approach and the most useful exercises, since as a relative you may well be needed later to help the patient with them after they've returned home.

Other members of the team appear later.

I looked on while she first watched Dilys totter up and down the ward, and then gave her a zimmer to use, before escorting her back to bed.

A zimmer is a lightweight metal frame with four legs, used to help people with walking difficulties. There are various designs.

"You'll have to get one of those for me to use when I'm back home," Dilys said, sounding worried.

I tried to make light of it. "No problem – we'll get one for every room."

The masses of flowers from friends and relations that crowded the bedside and spilt over on to the windowsill were a sign of the affection in which she was held. But sadly, the little treats of chocolates and grapes that had been brought remained untouched.

"I need the loo, Huw," she said. "Quick." I went to look for a nurse. In the office one was talking on the phone, but I caught another carrying a couple of sheets down the corridor. "Be along in a minute," she said.

I waited: no sign of the nurse. "I can't wait, Huw."

"I'll take you," I said. We staggered slowly down the ward to the toilet, where I had to help her on and off the loo. What a change in a fit, well person, I thought to myself, as I helped her back quietly to bed.

By now, I'd learnt that Dr. Feldman was a general physician, whose specialism was kidneys, and that most patients in the ward had kidney problems. I wondered if that was why the nurses hadn't been checking her fluid intake: she wasn't a kidney patient.

One of the key issues in getting the right diagnosis and treatment is being referred to the most appropriate consultant: medicine is now so very specialised that it's not always helpful to be sent to someone whose skills lie in a different field. Lay persons won't be aware of the local possibilities, but the GP will. Don't hesitate to ask him or her to discuss this with you. In this case I didn't, but the situation was complicated by it being an emergency admission, and the need to take any bed available.

It's quite common for relatives to wonder whether the patient is being seen by the right consultant. As a guide, stroke patients are usually seen by neurologists or (as in Dilys's case) by general physicians, or, if they're elderly, by geriatricians.

I felt I had to know what was going on, and waited until I caught one of the junior doctors coming round the ward.

"Oh yes," he confirmed, "Dilys's scan was quite clear, as were the blood tests."

"So what does Dr. Feldman think is wrong?" I asked.

"He thinks she has a virus," he replied. "It should work itself out in three or four months. We'll move her out to St. Michael's as soon as there's a bed for her there."

St. Michael's was a small cottage type hospital, well liked in the locality. We knew elderly friends who'd gone there for recuperation after broken limbs and strokes. I told Dilys about the diagnosis and impending move.

"Good," she said. "The sooner the better."

By the end of the week, there was an obvious change. She was using a wheelchair, now, instead of a frame, I noticed. To her shame she wet the bed while I was there. I fetched the nurses. They were quite cheerful as they changed the sheets. "Oh don't worry," one said. "Half the patients here have the same problem."

I could see how embarrassed she was, and felt despondency grip me briefly again.

Meanwhile, I tried to decode the diagnosis. Better in three or four months? That was a positive outcome, well worth the wait. Then doubts crept in. It didn't sound as if there was to be any treatment. And a virus? Anyone going to see a doctor with a mystery problem seemed to be diagnosed either with a virus or a trapped nerve, I thought. Here was my Dilys deteriorating visibly, day by day. Did they really know what was going on? I felt my anxieties rise. I really had to see the consultant.

It can be difficult to get access to the doctor in charge. Remember that he or she is a busy person, and you'll have to fit in with their schedule, no matter how busy you yourself may be.

There is no 'best way' of going about this. The consultant, like any doctor, owes a duty of confidentiality to the patient and no one else, and technically can only discuss the patient's case with another person with the patient's written consent. In practice, where the patient is seriously ill, the enquirer is a close relative with responsibilities for the patient, and consent can be assumed to be implicit, the doctor may decide to ignore this duty of confidentiality. (This happened on my first visit to the GP on Dilys's behalf.)

If the medical staff are willing to see you on these terms, one way of meeting the consultant is to ask the ward sister or ward manager. She may be helpful, and try to arrange a time.

Or she may suggest that you catch him or her during a ward round. This is not as easy as it sounds, since visitors are often excluded from the ward during consultants' rounds, and you are left to waylay the consultant as he or she exits from the ward. If Sister hasn't alerted him beforehand this may feel to him more like an ambush than a meeting.

Or you can get in touch with the consultant's secretary, preferably in writing, and ask for an appointment. This may mean that you'll have to wait: to save a little time drop the letter in the secretary's office. Having a friendly word with the secretary when you call can help.

But stick at it: you have a right to see the doctor in charge.

Second week of June

I remembered it was a Saturday. I'd have to wait until after the weekend before seeing Dr. Feldman, so I bottled up my anxieties, and concentrated on the two visits to Dilys each day. The daily routine of meals and household chores seemed to slip past without notice, though throughout the summer I was often invited to eat with friends, a wonderful kindness. Quite apart from not having to cook myself, these meals gave the quiet pleasure of chatting with other couples living in unstressed normality, the chance to catch up on the trivia of living in our little community, and the opportunity to talk to others about Dilys's situation. All this helped to release some of the anxieties and to relax me.

When someone asks how things are, it's so easy to put a bold face on it and say something neutral, like 'Oh we're managing thanks,' or something factual, like 'She's going to be moved in a few days' time.' Call it counselling, talk therapy, whatever you will: seize the chance to discuss your own worries. Others have often been through similar situations and understand your situation better than you realise. They want to know how you are doing, and since 'a little fellow feeling makes us wondrous kind', they can sometimes offer simple practical suggestions, like the friend who suggested that Dilys might like some of her personal scent brought in – which indeed she did. More importantly, the chance of sharing your feelings with others is helpful to you. There's no need to be concerned that you may be boring your friends; you'll soon sense if you are.

Another simple point, but well worth emphasising: never turn down any invitation. Don't worry about being a burden, or taking advantage of the kindness of friends and neighbours, and certainly don't think about having to repay invitations at a difficult time. Just say 'Yes please.'

The weekend was mixed. The good news was that both the sons came to see their mother, one from Bristol and the other from near Birmingham. They'd arranged to come in on different days, so Dilys had a real family weekend, and her pleasure showed. She wanted to hear all the news of their families, particularly her grandchildren, and she really enjoyed the photographs they brought of their recent holiday together.

But her speech was definitely poorer. Dilys always spoke very clearly and intelligibly, but now her sentences were shorter, she had difficulties getting them out, and sometimes stumbled over words. The two boys had visited the previous weekend and both now noticed a difference, and although the virus diagnosis reassured them, they were glad I was going to see Dr. Feldman as soon as possible.

After both boys had left, and before I went home, she took my hand in hers, and suddenly said,

"I do feel strange. Do you think I'm dying, Huw?"

The question hit me like a hammer blow. I'd never considered that possibility. The GP had certainly mentioned that she might have a serious condition, but she was now in hospital, getting skilled investigations – no one here had said anything other than that this might be a three month illness. I had to reassure her.

"Of course not. You're going to St. Michael's for recuperation, and then we'll get you home again: as soon as possible, too."

I smiled cheerfully, sat with her until after the allotted time, and tried to talk with her about the children's news. But she was quiet and introspective, thinking her own thoughts, trying to come to terms with her steady deterioration, I felt. I gave her a specially warm kiss before I left for home. Her question had disturbed me.

Back at home I returned to the daily chores. This housework is really not too difficult, I thought. Just a weekly swish round with the hoover, and that's the cleaning. Anyone who's ever had a camping holiday would find a modern stove a doddle, and with ready meals – why cooking's easy, though it's a bit boring to have to do it every day. And a weekly wash? No problem with the washing machine: that's easy too. Then my hubris, my pride, took a serious knock. I suddenly remembered I hadn't emptied the tumble-dryer; the clothes had been lying there for two days. No point in trying to hang up the twisted pile that emerged. Better do them again. Perhaps there was more to think about than I'd realised.

On Monday I went straight to Dr. Feldman's secretary. She shared a small office with three other medical secretaries. They all seemed quite surprised to see a visitor; I guessed all non-staff contact was usually made by phone, but I've always found a personal contact more effective.

"He's away ill," she said. "He'll be off work all week."

I felt cross; why did he have to be off work when I needed to see him so urgently? This was irrational, I realised. But I still felt frustrated.

"But I can make an appointment for Dr. Simmons, if you like," the secretary said. "She's taking on Dr. Feldman's work while he's away."

We fixed an appointment for a couple of days' time.

An appointment is likely to be short, so it's important to make the most of it. It's useful to make a list of the questions that you want to ask, and take it with you. You will want to mull over the answers later, so try to make a brief note of the key facts and opinions as they are given. Time makes it easy to forget or distort matters, so it's often helpful to expand the summary immediately afterwards when the discussion is fresh in your memory.

Back in the ward, Dilys was waiting expectantly for me, sitting in the bedside chair in which the nurses had placed her, the headphones, on which she liked to listen to the radio, hanging uselessly beside her; she couldn't put them on. As at every visit she wanted me to get her back into bed. This was a struggle, since she was so weak, and I had to call the nurses to help. I didn't want to bother them over such a simple procedure, but they didn't want me to help – you might hurt yourself, they said. They were reluctant to have her back in bed, too, but I couldn't resist her appeals, she was so pale faced and helpless.

Back in bed, she suddenly kissed me very warmly and at length. For several minutes she covered me with kisses, something she'd not done before. She didn't want to let me go.

What did this mean? It was as if she was going away, saying goodbye before a long journey. I thought of the previous evening, when she asked about dying. Perhaps she knew more about her condition than any of us did. I didn't know what to say, so I said nothing.

There was no improvement showing. She still wasn't eating and drinking, had no bladder control, her speech was poorer, as was her vision. She was feeling more tired still. The only positive point was that she complained much less of pain in the right side of her head.

Most stroke patients feel tired after a stroke. Pain too is a common feeling – understandably, since they will probably have lost some movements. But there are different kinds of pain, and it's always worth ensuring that the doctor knows how the patient feels. Both problems, pain and tiredness, usually improve after a few months of recovery.

Dr. Simmons was a small, dark haired lady, quiet and soft spoken. There was an open file on her desk – Dilys's I assumed. She waved me to a seat beside her while she explained that she hadn't seen Dilys herself, but had all her notes. She confirmed that the brain scan was entirely clear, apart from a small amount of atrophy round the periphery – entirely normal in someone of Dilys's age (she was 76). I asked about the general deterioration, which worried me so much. "It could be that the blood supply to the brain is affected," she said. She agreed that Dr. Feldman's diagnosis was that it was a virus. I pressed her.

"What virus is it?" I asked.

"We don't know that. But the best line for Dilys is to go to St. Michael's, where they have an excellent physiotherapy department."

"If there's no specific diagnosis, can I have her home?"

"Much better for her to have a week or two at St. Michael's first. The rehabilitation there is excellent."

I thanked her for her time – she'd given me a good 20 minutes, and after all Dilys wasn't her patient.

Dilys was delighted to learn that the move to St. Michael's was definitely on. "The sooner the better," she said.

That evening the GP rang to ask how we were getting on. I told her about the virus diagnosis and my unease about it. There was a pause.

"Sometimes we do use that diagnosis if we're not sure what the real problem is," she said. "I've done it myself."

"I thought so. I just wish they'd told me that openly." Then I told her about the move to St. Michael's for physiotherapy.

"Excellent," she said. "Dr. Phillips is the consultant geriatrician; there's no one better."

A geriatrician? Dilys, the bright lively lady, the first rate bridge player, the life and soul of so many parties, a geriatric case? Another sickening blow, another adjustment to make.

While physiotherapists work in general hospitals, small local hospitals are often used as 'stroke centres', where the teams of professionals who collaborate in the recovery and rehabilitation of stroke patients are based. Referral to one of these centres is a normal and advantageous procedure, since they usually offer more intensive help than can be provided in a general hospital.

Third week of June

No doctor had seen Dilys for days.

"They come and see the other patients," she said.

It was as if they'd washed their hands of her while they waited for a bed at St. Michael's. I tried to prick the little bubble of anxiety I felt, telling myself that if the doctors weren't worried, it must be a good sign, but the bubble kept returning. She was usually in the chair when I arrived, and she always pointed to the bed, pleadingly. Although the ward was warm, she felt cold, and I went to search for a blanket, not always easy to find.

If she was in bed, the sheets were often wet, though when I called the nurses, they were cheerful and uncomplaining about changing her and the sheets. Washing nighties was often a twice-a-day routine now.

She was looking forward to St. Michael's: she knew it from visiting friends who'd been there, and liked it.

By midweek she'd been padded up to save the washing. The nurses were often busy when she wanted to be changed, so I took her to the toilet and changed her myself. I soon had no scruples about a male in the female loo; no one seemed to object. But her ability to use a zimmer had now gone, and it was a question of manoeuvring her in and out of a wheelchair for the little journey to and fro. Not easy, but I soon learnt.

Handling a wheelchair properly requires a little skill – easy to learn, but worth learning. Managing the brakes and footrests, descending a small drop correctly, for example, are simple techniques that just need a little practice if you're not used to chairs. There's usually someone about who's experienced and ready to give help, and it's sensible to ask for it.

On Friday, her bed was empty. Her chair was unoccupied. Where was she?

"Oh Mr Watkins, we rang this morning and left a message on your answering machine. Dilys has gone to St. Michael's."

I thanked Staff Nurse and drove off to find Dilys. I didn't feel the gratitude I should have felt for the fortnight spent in the care of the hospital.

St. Michael's was about 15 miles away, a pleasant drive through quiet countryside to the little market town. The hospital itself was a small, modern, red brick building, approached by a drive through green lawns. It was a single storey building, a square surrounding a small courtyard. From each side of the square, glass doors opened into the courtyard, where brick paths led past seats and through small flowerbeds. It was a sunny day, and the whole impression was pleasing.

The reception secretary waved me on, through the lobby, until I saw Sister sitting behind a big desk, which commanded two small wards. Sister was a tall lady, early forties, I thought. I was struck by her very dark eyes, so dark that when she looked at you it seemed as if they were without pupils, just two black discs in the eye sockets. Her hair was even darker, black as a raven, drawn back in a severe bun that accentuated her pleasant, alert face. I later learnt that the hospital was divided in two for administration, with a different Sister in charge of the wards in each half. I could see Dilys in bed in one of the four bedded wards. It was light and airy, with big windows. Sister smiled.

"Of course you can see her," she said. "And there's no set visiting time. Come when you want to."

I suddenly felt happier.

Hospitals have personalities, which vary from hospital to hospital, and indeed from ward to ward within each hospital. A visitor can sense and feel this almost immediately. While there may not be much difference in the medical procedures that similar hospitals offer, one that offers a warm, welcoming approach makes an enormous difference to the quality of the recovery a patient makes. And a stroke patient, so often feeling tired and depressed at the sudden loss of functions, needs this as much as any patient. As with other institutions, the tone of a hospital depends heavily on the leadership, and while there is little a visitor can do to influence this, it's never amiss to try to reinforce the hospital's attitude by expressing your appreciation for it where appropriate.

Dilys was pleased to see me. There was no media station, I noticed, and I resolved to buy a portable radio so that she could listen to her favourite station. Music was one of her loves. In the early days of our relationship my rival had been a music student, and he'd nearly won. He had long since disappeared, but her long standing love of music had not been lost. We'd been to many concerts together, mainly classical, but also pop and jazz, for her taste was catholic. She'd want Classic FM, I was pretty sure of that.

Some patients prefer radio to television; lying back, eyes closed, listening to a favourite programme is less demanding than watching. It's worth checking the earphones provision. Other patients may prefer the television programme, and won't want to be distracted by the music your relative likes.

Now what was going to happen to her here? She didn't know, but didn't seem worried about it. Sister looked very approachable, so I walked over and asked her.

"Better see the doctor," she said. "He's on his rounds, but he'll be back here before long." I soon saw an elderly man in a white coat standing by the desk outside, chatting to Sister. He looked like the doctor, so I went out and plunged straight in, asking what was really wrong with Dilys.

The doctor explained in a surprisingly soft voice that he was a locum, standing in for the senior registrar who normally looked after the little hospital, but was away for the day. He examined a file, a very fat one, I thought. He turned the pages.

"Strange," he said. "There's no actual diagnosis, but I see she's been depressed." My heart sank again. Still on that old trail! I shook my head.

"I'm sure there's something much more wrong than that."

"Dr. Dayala will see her tomorrow," he said, "We'll do nothing today, she needs a day or so just to settle down."

Before leaving I went for a short walk through the little hospital, down the corridor, past the kitchen, until I came across a large room, small tables and dining chairs at one end, comfortable armchairs at the other. Some half dozen patients in dressing gowns were watching television.

"Bob!" I exclaimed. An old friend was sitting in a wheelchair by one of the tables, a plate of sandwiches and tea in front of him. Bob was in his eighties, a widower I'd met years ago through a charity committee. "What are you doing here?"

His answer was unintelligible. He saw my puzzlement and used one arm to point to the uselessness of the other. He tried to reply again. This time, guessing from his gestures, I was able to translate the heavily slurred words.

"I've had a stroke."

It's difficult to keep up a one-sided conversation. But if you don't try, the stroke patient feels more isolated than ever. Keep talking, even if he or she can't reply, or if the reply is hard to follow. Don't let them relapse into feeling disengaged from the normal world of human intercourse; this can reinforce feelings of depression. Most stroke patients can hear you, and want to hear you. Mike Ripley's book, *Surviving a Stroke* (see back of book for details), deals with the experiences of stroke patients and is well worth reading.

I took in the obvious signs of lost movement down one side and the damaged speech. These were the conventional signs of the common image of stroke victims. This is different from Dilys, I thought: Bob may have problems, but at least he's eating, and talking, too, after a fashion. I managed to grasp that he'd been in St. Michael's a week.

"Would you like a wheel around?" I asked, thinking that he was probably wheeled from bed to lounge to therapy and nowhere else. So after he finished his tea I took him for a brief tour of the hospital, out to the courtyard and around the corridors before returning him to the lounge, and promising to see him again.

When patients are well enough, they often like a change of scenery. Hospital staff are usually too busy with essential activities, but relatives and friends can enhance their visits by offering patients the chance to see something different from the confines of the daily routine.

When I arrived the next day Dilys was having physiotherapy. At last, something positive was happening. Two very pleasant physiotherapists and a nurse were trying to persuade her to walk a couple of steps to her bedside chair, using a frame.

"Come on Dilys, you can do it," they urged. They looked at me as if I could help. I joined the chorus of encouragement. "Just move that foot forward a little, my love, and then sit on the chair." The foot remained fixed firmly to the floor.

"Come, on, just try a little harder." I saw the look of desperation on Dilys's face. I felt a great surge of pity for her. Of course she was trying hard. Trying with all her might. It wasn't that she wouldn't move the foot; she couldn't. This was almost cruelty. I shook my head to the physios.

"She can't do it," I said sadly. Walking, that skill we learn as babies, that had gone; would it ever come back? They put Dilys back into bed.

It is difficult for stroke patients to recover immediately the functions that have been lost. As far as movement is concerned, the intention to move the limbs is as strong as before, as are the muscles involved in the movement. The problem is that the ability to translate intention into action has been damaged by the stroke: the brain cannot convey the message. The frustration at being unable to carry out what had often been the simplest of actions is a very depressing experience, and the right balance of sympathy and encouragement is needed from relatives as well as professionals.

I had a chat with Sister before I left.

"We're a little concerned about the eating, or rather the not eating." she said, "So we've arranged for the speech therapist to do a swallowing test." My spirits rose again. They were trying to do something.

There were three nice ladies in the ward, and I went to chat with them while Dilys was being wheeled to the toilet. One explained that the nurses had been putting Dilys to sit in her wheelchair, but that it had been uncomfortable for her, since she couldn't rest her head. So they'd moved her to an armchair by the window, where she rested much more comfortably on cushions. Good, I thought again. The nurses are thinking about her needs.

"Dilys waves to us in the mornings, though she doesn't say anything," the lady went on. Doesn't or can't, I thought to myself. Was speech the next skill to go? At least she's trying to communicate, I thought, trying to find a shaft of hope.

Next, the occupational therapist sought me out. She was pleased that we lived in a bungalow.

"You'll probably need a few modifications and extra facilities when Dilys comes home, even though it's a bungalow," she said. "I'll come to the house to advise. I'll make an appointment later on when we know more about Dilys's condition and needs."

I learnt that the hospital prided itself on its ability to return patients to care in the home. This was looking positive: when Dilys returned I was going to get a lot of help.

Occupational therapists, like the speech therapists mentioned earlier, are members of the team working with stroke victims. The occupational therapists help with the devices that some patients may need to cope with everyday living – cooking, washing, etc. In addition they advise over any modifications (e.g. support rails, ramps for steps) to the house that make it easier to get around. They can also suggest activities for patients who may be bored by the new limitations on their normal interests.

More news! Janet rang to say she'd booked a flight and was coming over in three or four days. I suggested she waited to see how her Mum progressed before making all the arrangements with her husband for the care of the children, but our daughter was adamant – the flight was booked and she was coming. I felt very cheered.

When I told Dilys, her eyes lit up in way I hadn't seen for a few days.

"It's such a long flight for her," she managed to croak out. "More than 40 hours door to door."

I nodded: her mind was still sharp.

It's really important for children to make the effort to visit the parent. Cards and phone calls are helpful, but nothing lifts both the patient and the partner as much as a visit.

Our older son visited again the following day. Dilys was as pleased as ever to see him. But then she held his hand.

"Tell me," she said, looking straight at John, and talking in what had become a deep, slurred voice, "Are you happy?"

I caught my breath. What a strange question, asked so seriously. What did it mean? Why did she want reassurance about her son's happiness? Was it a need to know that her child was enjoying the life she'd given him? And did she want to know now, because she felt she might soon not be able to ask the question?

By now her speech was indeed very difficult to understand. She spoke quietly, too, and to my astonishment she sometimes replied to questions in Welsh. That had been the language her parents must have used when she was a little girl, before the family moved to England, I remembered. Were the first words to come, the last to go?

Dilys was often sitting in the chair by the window, looking sleepy. Her speech had virtually gone. By chance, I was present when the speech therapist tried the swallowing test.

"Come on Dilys, try to move that tongue to help you swallow."

The therapist turned to me, shaking her head. "She can't do it."

"Will she regain it?" I asked.

I received the standard reply. "We can't say," she answered.

It was lunchtime. John was at the hospital and I was at home when the phone rang. The GP was calling.

"I've just heard from Dr. Dayala," she named the senior registrar at St. Michael's. "Dilys has had a brainstem stroke."

Many people think of a stroke as the sudden loss of the use of one side of the body, sometimes accompanied by loss of speech and drooping face muscles. If leg use is lost as well as arm use, then walking becomes very difficult. These are indeed fairly common effects, but far from the only ones. The key feature of a stroke is damage to the brain, to the complicated connections that control nearly all body functions. The effects of the stroke depend on where the damage occurs and how serious it is. Since the brain controls nearly all human functions, there are many different effects. And as I was to learn, while a brain scan usually shows the damage clearly, this is not always the case.

Last week of June

Stroke! It was the first time that word had been used since Dilys herself had used it when all this started. At last a diagnosis. My mind flashed to the various stroke victims I'd known, people with unintelligible speech, people unable to walk, people in wheelchairs...I thought of Bob. I'd been seeing him most days. He now was able to walk a few steps with the aid of a stick: his speech was still slurred, but definitely a little more intelligible. Bob had indeed been depressed, but depressed because of the stroke.

"I've fought and won a lot of battles in my life," he'd said at first, "but I'm going to lose this one." But latterly the shock at the sudden change in his life had begun to fade. His improvement was obvious, not least to Bob himself, and he was looking forward to going home next week. His attitude was much more positive. Was this the future for Dilys, too? When would she be coming home?

Would earlier diagnosis have helped Dilys? Yes in the sense that the right nursing care could have been started earlier, and she could have been made more comfortable from the start. No in the sense that the effects of a stroke are not immediately reversible, and initial recovery is gradual.

Much more can be done to prevent a stroke happening than to cure it. Once a person is known to be at risk, perhaps through having experienced a TIA, medication can be prescribed, and in some cases surgery might be suggested. So again, it really is important for the patient to be seen by a stroke specialist as early as possible.

John, our older son, was visiting Dilys that afternoon. It was a day when Dr. Phillips, the geriatric consultant, happened to be visiting St. Michael's, and John had managed to have a word with him.

John was impressed. "He's very clear and direct," he said. "He told me he was certain that Mum has had a brainstem stroke. But I'm afraid he also said that the future was very uncertain. He wouldn't make any predictions."

What's a brainstem stroke, I wondered.

Nearly all the nerves carrying messages to and from the brain pass through the brainstem, roughly at the base of the skull. It's as if all roads linking London to the North, East and West had to squeeze together through a narrow gap in the Chilterns. A major accident at that point could disrupt communications right across the country, much more than an accident in one of the districts of the capital.

So, to leave the metaphor, a stroke in the brainstem can affect nearly every function, including most muscular movements and most sensations.

I tried to absorb these two pieces of news: a brainstem stroke and a very uncertain future.

"He wants to send Mum over to the main hospital for a brainstem scan," John went on. "Apparently it's a different procedure from the ordinary scan. He wants to know whether there's bleeding going on."

Bleeding: what did that mean?

As mentioned earlier, one of the two main types of stroke is caused by bleeding. If it's still continuing, then it's likely that more damage will be done and more functions will be lost.

"I brought these leaflets from the hospital. They might be helpful," John said.

I took John to his train. When I got back home, I looked up brainstem stroke on the internet, and found a fairly simple site. It was clearly a very serious illness. One statistic leapt out: about 30% of brainstem strokes were fatal. Fatal! And Dr. Phillips, the specialist, had said the future was very uncertain. For the first time I began to contemplate a very black possibility. I felt shocked. But of course, if 30% were fatal, 70% were not: the probabilities were on our side. My spirits rose a little.

With my mind in a whirl, I glanced at the leaflets John had brought, picking out one that was aimed at relatives. "You'll find you'll be riding an emotional roller coaster," it said.

How true that phrase was for me, and doubtless for many others who have watched their loved ones trying to recover from an illness that could have devastating results – but might not. Where the victim is in hospital, and all the care is in the hands of others, there is little the rela-

tives can do, except watch, wear the mask of encouragement, and prepare for what might be very changed circumstances. Every relative of a
stroke victim must be prepared to live the hopes and fears of an uncertain future.

The following day I asked about seeing Dr. Phillips myself.

"He only consults here once a week," Sister said. "He'll be back
here next Tuesday, and by then we'll know a little more about
how Dilys is getting on. We'll arrange for you to see him then."

She went on to say that they were concerned about Dilys not
eating, and even more concerned about her fluid intake. They
were going to put a drip in.

I was concerned too, but very glad that they were dealing with
it. Dilys did look comfortable and relaxed in bed. Yet I noticed
that the portable radio I'd brought in was never being used.
Was switching it on, even that simple task, too much for her?

I saw Bob again in the day room. He was definitely being discharged in a few days' time. The physiotherapy and the exercises were effecting a steady improvement. "Dressing is difficult, though," he confided in his slurred voice.

We usually dress standing up, a habit that stroke victims often need to
unlearn, since balance is sometimes affected, and there is a danger of
falling. Sitting on the bed is often a better arrangement. Another issue is
dressing when the use of limbs may have been lost or limited. The choice
of clothing can make a difference to ease of dressing, e.g. velcro instead
of buttons, or snap-on fastenings. Some therapists believe in trying to

maximise the use of a damaged limb to get as much function returning as possible, while others think that it's more important to use the better limb, i.e. dressing at all costs. This is something to discuss with the nurse or the therapist.

The Disabled Living Foundation, listed on the White Ladder website, offers over 50 free leaflets covering advice and aids for dressing and many other activities such as bathing, eating, communicating, mobility, etc.

I left Bob, and returned home.

Back home, I was searching for something in Dilys's wallet when I came across the kidney donor card that she always carried. I recalled how strongly she felt about giving life to others. Some 20 years ago, when there'd been a campaign for kidney donors, she'd insisted on us both carrying cards. There was little point in the card staying in her wallet at home: if it were to be needed, it would be needed quickly. The obvious place for it would be the hospital, but perhaps that would be tempting fate. Could I ask her? No, that would be insensitive in the extreme. What would she want? She'd want it readily available, I was sure of that; so after a moment's reflection, I decided to take it to Sister, and handed it over with a feeling of apprehension at what I was doing. I didn't want to contemplate the circumstances in which the card would be needed. Sister accepted the card as if this was an everyday procedure, one that every patient followed. She was pleased that Dilys was a donor, and after explaining that the donor procedures were now more comprehensive, she filed the card with the case notes. I felt a little better.

The nurses were happier now that the dehydration was being relieved. I noticed that Dilys never asked for the loo now, in spite of having a good fluid intake. I wondered whether she was aware of bladder pressure, or whether that had gone too?

The appointment for the new scan would be in a fortnight's time. A fortnight! I wondered how crucial this procedure was. Any price was worth paying if it helped, so I asked about paying for a private scan.

"It won't make any difference at all," Sister said, "that's the earliest they can do it."

Meanwhile, Janet was on the plane, on her way to see her Mum. I remembered Dilys's black humour.

"Don't bother coming over to my funeral," she'd said to Janet, more than once. "I won't know whether you're there or not. You come and see me when I'm alive."

A couple of days later, I met Janet at the airport and drove her straight to the hospital, where she went in at once to see Dilys. Poor Dilys couldn't say anything, but there was no doubting the smile of recognition as Janet approached her bed. She hadn't seen Janet for more than a year, and it was worth everything to see that flash of pleasure, that familiar smile of happiness. I left mother and daughter obviously luxuriating – no other word for it – in each other's company, Janet telling her all the news about her grandchildren, and

Dilys nodding and smiling in acknowledgement. Nothing could cheer her up more, I thought.

Once again, visits from children can make a tremendous difference to a patient. Visits from other close relatives usually help too. But it's as well to be sure that the relative is one the patient wants to see!

Since she couldn't talk we tried to think of other ways of communicating. Writing of course! My handwriting is a family joke, an indecipherable scrawl, but Dilys had always written so clearly. I took a small board with a sheet of paper in to the hospital ward.

"Is there anything you'd like, Dilys?" I asked, and gave her a pencil. Her pencil traced a thin, wavery line on the paper: it was entirely meaningless. She was trying to say something, but couldn't make herself understood. Her neat handwriting had gone, replaced by something between a scrawl and a scribble; yet another skill lost, I realised sadly.

"Just a minute," Janet said, and on the board she drew two large letters, a Y and an N. "This is 'Yes', Mum," she said, "and this is 'No'. Now, is there anything you'd like?"

We watched as the hand moved slowly and shakily, the pointing finger resting clearly on the No. I felt a momentary pain. Was this the best communication Dilys could manage, when just six weeks ago speech was such a natural skill? Then a small gleam of hope lit up the darkening horizon before me: at least some communication had been restored.

Communicating with others is a basic human skill, but loss of speech doesn't always mean loss of communication. When speech is damaged, the first port of call is the speech and language therapist, who can help with the restoration of speech. Where speech has been permanently lost, there are various devices for helping the patient to convey wishes, to answer and ask questions; that is to communicate. At one end of the scale are simple boards with letters or symbols through which the patient can express thoughts. These are not to be underestimated: stroke victims have managed to write whole books using devices like these. At the other end of the scale are advanced technological aids, such as the electronic gadgetry used by the well known scientist, Stephen Hawking. Psychologists can be particularly helpful in working out the most suitable device for restoring communication, and like the speech and language therapists, they can be reached through the hospital or the GP.

Sister caught me. "We're still very worried about Dilys's weak state," she said. "We'll try nasal feeding over the weekend, instead of the drip. It means passing a feeding tube through her nose, straight down into her stomach," she explained.

They're doing all they can, I thought.

First week of July

Janet came with me again. I felt relaxed in her company, she was so bright and lively in spite of the circumstances. No need for me to worry about the household management now, she took it all over – what a pity she couldn't stay longer. But in far away New Zealand her husband was having to cope with his job, the house, and their children, and Janet had responsibilities there: she would have to return. Dilys would have approved of that decision – she had a strong moral sense, believing in doing the right thing, whether it was to her own advantage or not.

As we entered the hospital, Janet gave a cheery wave to Sister, sitting behind her desk in the spotless reception area. We walked into the ward. There was Dilys – but I couldn't see any nasal tubes. What did that mean? I held her hand for a few minutes, and then left mother and daughter together while I went to see Sister. She explained that they had tried nasal feeding twice, but each time Dilys had pulled the tube out.

"The nurses wanted to try again," she went on, "but I felt it was distressing Dilys too much."

I wondered how distressed poor Dilys had been. Then I thought again about her situation. I remembered how she had endured pain after past operations. She could always put up with discomfort, if it was necessary. I remembered how strong a character she was, and in my own mind I felt a dark suspicion forming. Had she pulled the tube out deliberately? Did she not want to be fed? Did she know what the hospital was trying to do and didn't want it? She had always insisted that she would never want to be kept going when life was pointless.

"I don't want to be a burden to anyone," she had said firmly.

That evening I shared my thoughts with Janet. We had a long discussion, and we were both of the same opinion. Janet told me that Dilys had once made her promise faithfully never to let her live on in a helpless, burdensome state. I was surprised: I hadn't known about the promise. For a moment I wondered whether Dilys had felt that I myself would not have been able to take such a tremendous decision, even though I knew her wishes. That decision time was approaching, and it was such a relief to have another family member to share the burden.

Now that Janet had arrived, Dilys had seen all her three children. I remembered her odd question to John; "Are you happy?" Reassured by the answer, knowing that all her children were well, was she trying to tell us that she wanted to be allowed to die? Dark suspicion hardened into black certainty. I resolved to tell Sister the following day.

Sister made no comment.

"We do genuinely find some patients can't manage nasal feeding," she said after a pause. "But I know Dr. Dayala would like to discuss this with you. She'll be free tomorrow."

Dr. Dayala was the doctor in day-to-day charge of the small hospital. The nurse who took me to her consulting room clearly liked her. "A very nice lady indeed," she told me. She turned out to be a pleasant Asian woman, small and round, with a gentle manner, though her heavily accented English was not always easy to understand. She sat behind a large desk, metal rimmed spectacles perched on her nose, the nurse on a chair beside the desk.

"Since your wife can't take the nasal feeding, we'll have to try feeding through a peg in the stomach," she explained.

Peg in the stomach? What did that mean? Yet another new situation to face. She must have seen my worried expression.

"It's quite a simple operation," she went on, explaining the details. "We need to see how she responds to proper nutrition."

Feeding through a peg involves making a small opening in the stomach to allow a tube to pass directly into it. The tube is attached to a feeding bottle that holds a nutritious liquid. This enables the patient to receive food directly, instead of through the normal route. It sounds a worrying operation, but is in fact a fairly routine procedure.

I had to put to her what I thought – no, knew – would be Dilys's wishes.

"I am absolutely sure that my wife would not want this, doctor."

"We can't deprive our patients of food," she said, still kindly. "While patients are in our care we must do our best to feed them."

The nurse must have sensed my resistance, and immediately supported her. "It would be very wrong to let Dilys die. Dr Dayala would be in trouble with the medical authorities."

I tried again. "Dilys has been a lively, lovely lady, active all her life. She's 76. Suddenly, she's hardly able to speak or communicate in any way; she can't eat, taste or swallow; she's bed bound – no mobility at all. She has no bladder or bowel control; she can't see. After over 50 years of marriage I know her wishes so well. She would not want to go on living in this condition. She would want to leave us as smoothly and as painlessly as possible."

The doctor tried another tack. "But there is always hope, always the chance that the clot will dissolve with time. So apart from the legal requirement, there are good medical reasons to carry on feeding."

For a moment I thought of Bob. But his improvement had been palpable, slow maybe, but definite. He was regaining mobility and speech: he seemed to have retained all other functions. He was particularly pleased that the awkward use of bedpan and bottle, a major source of embarrassment to him as to so many stroke patients temporarily confined to bed, was no longer needed. But Dilys was deteriorating every day: it was so different.

Most stroke patients, like Bob, respond to the treatment plan. Physiotherapy helps the gradual recovery of movement; speech therapy helps the gradual recovery of speech. The other support services – occupational therapist, social worker, etc. – are introduced as usual when the need arises. No one can guarantee a complete recovery, but most patients make a gradual improvement, usually over a long period, perhaps a year or more.

In the quiet room the remorseless debate continued. I found it hard to believe that the lost functions could be miraculously restored. The two people opposite were pleasant, but adamant, trying hard to convince me that it was their duty to their patient. As a final shot the doctor added that the alternative, leaving her on water only, would mean that she would suffer hunger pains. Did I want that for her?

I wanted what she would want, but I was in no position to argue with two experts who believed they were doing their best for my wife. While Dilys was their patient, they felt it was their duty to feed her. I bowed to the inevitable. I left the room overwhelmed by a feeling of disbelief: who would have thought a couple of months ago that I would have been sitting in a strange, small room, calmly arguing for my lovely wife's death? Yet I felt unhappy; by acquiescing to the ethics of the medical profession, I'd somehow let Dilys down. My emotions were in turmoil.

It can be argued that the closer we approach death, the more we cling to life, any sort of life, overriding any previous views. Yet how many of us would want to leave this life as a "drugged, unconscious patient, full of tubes for breathing, eating and elimination, a subhuman object for manipulation by the medical technicians"?*

Decision on this difficult situation only arises for a minority of stroke victims, those where hope is absent and where the patient's wishes are clearly known. Where it does arise, the relatives are faced with heart-rending decisions. So too are the medical staff, having to steer a route between a rock and a hard place, the demands of medical ethics on one hand, and the wishes of the patient and relatives on the other. Every case is different, and for most stroke victims (like Bob) skilled treatment and encouragement can result in a quality of life that, although different, is still well worth living.

The next day we had an appointment with the social worker, arranged a week previously. Alison was a gentle, kindly lady, large and matronly, and with the kind of reassuring voice that calmed her clients. She explained the hospital's target of placing patients into care at home, and wanted to discuss the arrangements for Dilys. The wheel turned again; frustration began to ease. Did she know something I didn't? Were they really expecting Dilys to recover? Should I start to hope for the unbelievable?

I remembered the promise I'd given Dilys on that day the

*Neil Elliot in *The Gods of Life*.

ambulance took her to hospital. "Yes, once they've found out what's wrong, of course you'll come home." How I would love to be able to fulfil that promise. Could I really expect to have her sitting in her favourite window seat once again, looking out across the valley to the mountains she'd walked so often?

I heard Alison's voice mingling with my thoughts, as if I were tuned in to two radio stations at the same time. She was continuing with the practicalities. Yes, an hour's nursing, morning and evening, would be provided to help me. If I felt I needed more help this could be bought privately or from social services. We discussed the pros and cons; social services would be better; all their nurses had guaranteed qualifications, and there would be back-up should any nurse be unable to come.

We moved on to facilities. Yes, the occupational therapist would call to look at the home arrangements, and arrange for any modifications to be made. In my mind I was already moving a bed into the lounge, and wondering whether the door would need turning.

Alison continued. A hoist would be sent, and I would be given training in using it. I felt a tremor of apprehension. I'd seen the nurses struggling with hoists in the hospital; could I manage on my own? Alison sensed my uncertainty.

"Don't worry – you'll get some training in using it" she said.

Any other equipment needed would be provided, she went on. But none of this would be started until it was time for Dilys to leave hospital.

"What about this stomach peg?" I asked.

"Oh you'll be shown how to handle that, too."

I now had to grasp a new set of possibilities: somehow I had never considered Dilys coming home as a handicapped person. With a shock, I saw my life changing completely. At 76, I would have a new role as a carer, and there would be adjustments to make, major adjustments. So many freedoms and activities I took for granted would have to go. I'd be concentrating on caring for Dilys.

On the way home, Janet and I talked about the meeting. Familiar procedures for the hospital, we thought; they knew what they were doing. I tried to come to terms with the new situation.

The social worker is another member of the stroke team, working closely with the speech and language therapist and the occupational therapist. She knows what help the social service department of the local authority can provide, and is the link between it and the hospital.

The social services are there to help. They will probably contact you, but if not, it's really important to contact them yourself, perhaps through the GP or direct. There are so many different sources of support, and they are the experts in putting you in touch with them. Financial help, nursing help, help through local groups of fellow-carers – the social services provide the best channel through which these resources can be tapped in the first instance.

The following day was the day for the stomach peg. The operation would be done in the general hospital, about an hour's drive away. I would travel in the ambulance with Dilys, while Janet met us there.

Nine in the morning, and Dilys was ready, bundled up in a cocoon of blankets and strapped on to a trolley. I sat with her, holding her hand. This can't be doing her much good, I thought, as the ambulance bumped its way round the byroads, picking up patients in rural villages, and she lay there motionless, eyes closed. It took two hours to reach the hospital. The cheerful ambulance men carried her up to the waiting area for surgery. There were six or seven other patients waiting, and Janet went off to find some coffee for us. By one o'clock Dilys was still waiting, and we found some sandwiches. As ever, nothing for Dilys, lying asleep, the drip on its stand functioning quietly.

"Won't be too long now," the busy theatre nurse said. I wondered what Dilys was thinking. Was she suffering, lying there?

At two o'clock I signed the consent form, and she went in. I accompanied her into the theatre, marvelled briefly at the bright lights and the computer monitors, and returned to the recovery room to wait. I recognised some of the faces I'd seen waiting for surgery, lying on the beds, some awake, others still under anaesthetic. The nurses were checking each patient to confirm that they were ready to leave. Then Dilys was wheeled out of theatre. As she was lifted on to a recovery bed, I noticed the tube leading under her blanket. The nurse came over to chat, finding how much I knew about stomach pegs.

"Nothing at all," I confessed.

"You'll find it's best cleaned with Coke," she advised, going off to see to another patient. Coke? I felt bemused. How did I take it out of her stomach, what did it look like and how did I clean it? I needed to be shown it, to have a demonstration of what to do. What came to mind was the old Chinese proverb:

"I hear, and I forget; I see, and I remember; I do, and I learn.

An hour went by, then two. Dilys lay there, breathing quietly, eyes closed. I began to wonder about an ambulance for her, but the nurse reassured me.

"We'll find one, don't worry."

She was now the only patient left in the recovery room. I could see the staff gradually disappearing. Then a doctor came in.

"Hallo," he nodded at me. "I'm the surgeon. She's taking a bit of a time to come round, is she?"

I nodded. He leant down to her ear. "Dilys" he bellowed. Her eyes flickered momentarily, and he turned to the nurse.

"She can go."

We had the ambulance to ourselves, and it took us straight back to the little hospital, where Janet was waiting. It was after six o'clock, more than nine hours since Dilys had left, and the night staff were now on duty. The nurses put her back into her bed while Janet and I waited.

As the nurses tucked her up, I noticed a tremble. The tremble became more violent, until she started to shake, and the staff nurse came to help. By now Dilys was having difficulty in breathing; she was struggling, struggling so hard. I was very concerned: so were the nurses. They drew the curtains round the bed, and put her on oxygen, as I felt another downward swoop of the roller coaster.

No one can predict when the situation takes turns for the worse or turns for the better, but changes will occur, and being aware that they are likely, helps to meet them when they arrive. The important principle is not to be overwhelmed by moments like this; treatment for stroke patients does not always proceed smoothly.

The breathing eased a little, but wasn't right: we were still worried, and so clearly was Staff Nurse. She sent for the GP on night call. The struggle continued, while we anxiously waited out the half hour till he came, black medical bag in hand. He examined Dilys briefly, and advised continuing the oxygen.

After a while she seemed to settle. Staff Nurse came to check.

"Seems better," she said. "But we won't start feeding till the morning."

Janet and I prepared to go, when suddenly the struggle started again. Staff Nurse rang the doctor again, but he said there

was no point in him coming, he really couldn't do any more –
just continue the oxygen. We waited by the bedside, helpless.
At last the struggle for breath seemed a little easier, and Dilys
started to settle again.

"Would you like to stay the night?" Nurse asked me. "We have
a room for visitors, just down the corridor."

Janet went home, while I rested on the convertible bed in the
visitors' room. Each time I went to see Dilys, she was sleeping
peacefully.

"You get some sleep," said the nurse. "I promise to wake you if
anything changes."

What a day it had been, I thought, as I lay down on the couch.
There was Dilys, now apparently sleeping soundly, just a few
yards away from me. It was our first night under the same
roof since that morning, two months ago, when she left in the
ambulance. I fell into a deep sleep, feeling strangely comfort-
ed at spending a night so close to her.

In the morning, the crisis was over. Dilys was still sleeping
peacefully, and there was a feeding bottle hanging beside her
bed. The tube led beneath the bedclothes and into her
stomach. The nurses looked happier.

"She's getting some food now," Nurse said.

That afternoon Richard, my medical cousin, came to see Dilys.
He understood the situation at once, and sympathised with us
and with her. Although he felt the medical team had to do

what they were doing, his view was clear, and he recited the old couplet, succinctly advising doctors of their principles:

"Thou shalt not kill; but needst not strive
Officiously to keep alive."

"In Dilys's condition, I see little point in trying to prolong her suffering," he said, "knowing, as we all do, what her own attitude is. The best hope for her is that she gets a chest infection, quite likely after a long stay in bed in a weak condition. Many doctors wouldn't feel obliged to treat it with antibiotics, and that would give her the ending she wants, without doing violence to medical ethics."

He came with Janet and me to see Dr. Dayala that afternoon. For me, it was a less emotional discussion than before; I was now familiar with the arguments on both sides. Dr. Dayala repeated her view.

"I can't leave Dilys to starve," she said, and we agreed that we understood her position.

Richard raised the medical point. "If she gets an infection, a pneumonia, would you feel you had to treat her, or would you agree it might be kinder not to interfere, to save her going through the illness again?"

Dr. Dayala knew what she'd do. "I treat once, maybe twice, and then I consider leaving her untreated, if I felt there was no hope for the patient."

That was the best we could expect. It seemed a reasonable attitude.

This issue of keeping patients alive when their condition is agreed to be hopeless is a general issue, not limited to patients who have had a severe stroke, and is associated with the wider debate about euthanasia. It's a sensitive issue, on which strong views are held on both sides.

Second week of July

The following morning, Dilys was still sleeping, though she looked pale. Sister called me over. She told me that Dilys had regurgitated the feed, and was clearly unwell. What a rotten few days she'd had, I thought; even the liquid sustenance through the stomach peg was too much for her.

Sister went on. "We've decided to replace the food with water only," she said. I felt a mixture of relief and a great sinking of my spirit. It looked as if Dilys's wishes, and our wishes for her were being met adventitiously; she was now on water only since she couldn't manage food anyway. I sat by her bedside, trying to absorb the consequences. This would be the end, and I had to come to terms with it. Hopefully, it would be a dignified end.

Janet and Richard came in the afternoon, and we talked over the new development. I tried to remember stories of mountaineers left without food, living on water only. How long did they last? Was it three weeks? Six weeks? But they were fit people. On the other hand they were exposed to horrible weather conditions, while Dilys was getting wonderful care.

"It'll be weeks," said Richard, "but no one can say how many."

That evening, the three of us decided to eat at a local restaurant; something to take our minds off the drama being played out at the hospital. Beforehand, I rang the two boys, and told them of the new decision. Both were unhesitating. "It's what Mum would have wanted," they said.

Dilys was very quiet now. She smiled when we visited, so she certainly recognised us and could show pleasure. Her speech had virtually gone, though just occasionally she was able to offer a recognisable word. Odd grunts and other strange sounds emerged as she tried so hard to talk to us. My sadness at her plight was coloured by an overwhelming admiration for her: never once did she show distress at the condition she was in; no tears, no signs of misery at the frustration she must have been feeling.

The following morning Richard went home, and I went in to visit Dilys as usual. Dr. Dayala wanted to see me.

"Now that Dilys has settled after the operation we'll be starting to feed her again," she announced. I felt as if I'd been hit a sickening punch: my world swung round. Just after getting adjusted to what I'd imagined would be the gentle death that Dilys would have wished, just after Sister had taken the feeding away and put her on water, now she was being dragged back into life. What sort of life, and to what purpose? The speechless, incontinent, immobile person in the hospital bed wasn't the Dilys I knew, nor the Dilys she wanted to be. I needed time to adjust to this new situation. I thought quickly.

"It's definitely not what she would have wanted," I said, "and all the family can endorse that."

"But we don't know for sure that it was her wish. And even if she had written something while she was able to do so, we would not necessarily have followed it. People change their minds."

I remembered again the old adage: the closer to death the more one clings to life. But Dilys was not one to change her mind. She was a strong character, someone who stuck to her guns, someone who hated being a burden on anyone.

"But what kind of future will she have?" I asked.

Dr. Dayala offered hope. "Look," she said, "I've seen people in your wife's condition recover, and walk out of this hospital. We must try."

"I would like to consult with the family," I pleaded.

Dr. Dayala agreed. "But tell them fairly that I can't let a patient of mine starve to death," she said, "and you must come back quickly because Dilys is weakening."

I didn't stay long that morning, but gave Dilys a specially big hug before returning home and telling Janet about the new situation. That afternoon, after Janet had visited, we started phone calls. I began with the two boys, who were unanimous.

"It's not what Mum would have wanted."

How could I challenge the decision? I needed advice, and the best advice on how to challenge a medical decision would be a friendly doctor, I thought. I was on good terms with the doctors in our local practice, and so I rang the Health Centre. The GP whose advice I particularly wanted, an open, approachable doctor, sensible and friendly, was seeing patients, but the receptionist promised he'd call back.

The call came later that evening. The GP was as clear as I hoped he'd be. He reinforced what I was learning about hospitals, that hospitals were very strict about having to feed patients.

"It's a little different at home," he said. "I know your wife and I know the family, and if she were at home we might well just keep her on water, and let her fade away gently."

"What about the starvation pain that Dr. Dayala mentioned?" I asked.

"We could handle that with a pain driver." He mentioned the technical details.

At this point I suddenly felt overwhelmed by the poignancy of discussing the death of my life's partner in such a matter-of-fact way. Janet saw my distress, and took over the conversation. She did so brilliantly. I heard her asking about the likelihood of the recovery that Dr. Dayala had mentioned. I heard the answer, too.

"To be honest, if as you say she's been gradually deteriorating for eight weeks from a brainstem stroke, I'd say most unlikely."

The GP suggested that we could ask for another opinion, and gave the name of a neurologist who consulted at the hospital, before telling me to ring again if I wanted to.

Another old friend was a retired doctor, who knew Dilys and me well. To get another view I rang him too. He reinforced what I was rapidly learning about hospital ethics.

"They have to feed," he said. I asked him, too, about the chances of recovery.

"From what you tell me, very slim indeed. I'd say about 5% if you're lucky, and then how much recovery would you get?"

Finally, I rang Richard. He understood the dilemma very clearly, and as he knew Dilys so well I was relieved to hear him say that he would not have wanted to continue to feed her.

"But the decision to give up feeding is not an easy one for hospitals to take, and it's usually one that has to be taken at consultant level. So I'd advise you to see Dr. Phillips, her geriatric consultant. It would be courteous to mention to him any request you make for another opinion, too. Don't press him too hard over it," he went on. "There's no point in antagonising your consultant. If he seems reluctant to give up feeding, ask him about his views on treating the infections that will probably occur in patients in Dilys's condition."

Once again, always ask to see the consultant if you're concerned about treatment – but remember that they're busy professionals, there's no best way of getting access to them and you'll have to fit in to their schedules. But they really do hold the key to decisions on hospital patients.

The next day, Michael came over, and the three of us, Janet,

Michael and I went in to the hospital, three family members together.

It helps tremendously to have the support of family members, particularly children, when difficult meetings are to be faced. Not only is it reassuring for the immediate relative, but the hospital staff are more likely to pay attention to a united family team than to a single person.

Sister was of course our first port of call. I explained that the family was unanimous: we wanted Dilys to stay on water. My eyes filled with tears as I said it, but I just knew that it was the right decision for her.

Sister was very sympathetic. "But I can't override the doctors," she said. The impression I had was that she thought we were right, but that she was bound by the etiquette and rules of medical procedure.

"Dr. Dayala's not here today," she went on, "so I think you'd better see the senior Sister."

The three of us waited in the seminar room for the senior Sister, who'd ordered tea and biscuits for us from the kitchens.

She of course repeated the nursing view. Whatever they felt, they couldn't override the medical staff.

"How long can she live in this condition?" I asked. The Sister gave the stock answer. "No one can say."

I pressed her. "Would you say, from your experience, weeks, months, or years?"

"Oh I don't think it would be years."

"One year, would you say?"

"Unlikely to be a year, but no one can say. Everybody's different."

At last we had some sort of estimate; this stroke condition was unlikely to last more than a year, even with feeding.

Sister arranged a meeting with Dr.Dayala that afternoon, over at the main hospital where she was working.

At the risk of overemphasising things, all strokes are different. The Stroke Association states that a third of all stroke patients make a good recovery within a month, a figure well worth hanging on to. In Dilys's case, one of the key factors was the steady deterioration in her functions over a period of two months, not a good sign. Any sign of improvement in the first few weeks is good news for relatives of stroke victims.

Dr. Dayala was clear: she had to abide by medical procedures and feed Dilys.

Janet explained how torn she felt, remembering that she had solemnly promised her Mum years ago never to keep her going if ever she found herself in a helpless state.

"But we haven't her written wishes," Dr. Dayala said, "and even if we had she's in no state to confirm them."

I understood Dr. Dayala's point: she was implying that persons who are seriously ill, and close to death, sometimes change their previous views, and wish to cling to life. On the other hand, the reason for written wishes was precisely that they should be used when the writer was unable to communicate. I decided not to pursue the argument. I changed tack, and mentioned that we were thinking about asking for a neurologist's opinion. I felt a distinct hardening in Dr. Dayala's attitude.

"That won't help you at all. A neurologist will have no view on whether to feed a patient or not." The clear message was that feeding was the responsibility of the doctors in charge.

"What about treatment for an infection?" I thought it worth checking that she was still following the line she said she'd take when we'd seen her with Richard.

"She's already had one infection, which we treated successfully. If she has another, I might not treat, but it would depend on what's best for Dilys under the circumstances."

No promises, but no change either.

Before we went I thought I'd better tell her that I'd not yet seen Dr. Phillips, and would like to hear his opinion.

"Of course," she said. I felt Dr. Dayala was essentially a kind lady, humane, wanting to help Dilys within the limits of her view of medical ethics.

We went back to see Dilys later that afternoon, and then I asked Sister for an appointment to see Dr. Phillips.

"He's away for a fortnight's holiday," she said.

How could I convince the medical staff of Dilys's own wishes? The key was the consultant, Dr. Phillips. In preparation for his return from holiday, I decided to ask each of the children if they'd be willing to provide a written statement of what they understood their mother's wishes to be. Janet wrote hers before she left on the long flight back to her family; a strong statement, underlining her own feelings of failure at not being able to keep the promise she had made to her mother. Each of the two sons produced similar, independent statements. I wrote my own, and placed the four documents together, ready to show the consultant. No point in showing Dr. Dayala; I knew she would not be moved.

Be prepared for difficulties in seeing the consultant responsible for the care of patients. It would be marvellous if relatives could be treated like customers at a family store, where friendly staff are always available. But a hospital isn't like that: courtesy from staff should be expected, availability hoped for.

It was time for Janet's return flight.

"You need to get someone in to help you with the house, Dad."

"No, I can manage," I demurred.

"Yes you do; someone who does floors and loos once a week, and then anything else they have time for."

I listened to my daughter, had a word with a neighbour, and through her found Jean, who now comes in for two hours once a week. I find it a relief not to have to worry about the state of the house, the children feel happier knowing there's someone going in regularly, and it's company having someone working around the house. My friends in similar situations have all made similar arrangements. One has his ironing done by his help, another has his bed changed.

Help in the house at a time of stress is well worth thinking about. Some people find the routine of housework something that takes their mind off the worries of the illness, and may not like having someone else in their house. Others, the majority I think, find the chores yet another burden at a difficult time. If you can afford help, try it: neighbours can often suggest a reliable person.

Third week of July

Dilys had been moved. She was now in a side room for a single patient, a nice room with a view over the shrubs and paths of the courtyard. I felt another sinking of the heart. Perhaps the move made the nursing easier, but I remembered how, when my parents died, the move from the ward to a separate room was a signal that hope was fading. Dilys herself was as peaceful as ever, lying quietly, eyes closed, the gentle rise and fall of her chest as she breathed was the only sign of life. She seemed to be sleeping.

Was she conscious, I wondered? Was her mind active, and if so what was she thinking? She seemed unable voluntarily to move a muscle. I asked the nurses for their opinion.

"She does sometimes manage to open an eye slightly when we wash and change her in the mornings, but nothing otherwise," they said. "We move her position regularly to avoid any pressure sores: she herself can't do anything."

"Can you hear me, Dilys?" No response at all. I took her hand. Was that a slight pressure?

"If you can hear me, Dilys, squeeze my hand," I said.

Was that a slight return pressure? I tried again. No doubt about it; there was a slight answering pressure. So although all normal movement had gone, I could sense her tiny, feeble touch, like a fly landing on my palm. More importantly, she could hear me: there was still a conscious, living person inside that useless body. What was she thinking, I wondered again.

Post from Janet! She'd sent me a book, 'The Diving Bell and the Butterfly'.

What a strange title, I thought. When I read the outline, I realised its significance. The book was written by a Frenchman, Jean-Dominique Bauby, who'd suffered the same blow as Dilys, and was left with one movement only, in his case, the ability to move one eyelid. He'd retained this movement for over a year, and using it to respond 'yes' or 'no' to letters in an alphabet provided by friends, he'd 'dictated' the book letter by letter. It was only a short book, but what a triumph over difficulties!

I read and reread the book. He made it quite clear that inside a locked-in, motionless individual, was a living, feeling human being, one who spent the long hospital hours revisiting happy memories, imagining lost sensations of taste and touch and sight, thinking what he might do if only he were able to rejoin normal life. The title became clearer. The diving bell encapsulated his situation, cut off from the world, and the butterfly was his fluttering eyelid, his communication lifeline. Most importantly, the book made clear that in spite of being motionless, having lost so many functions, one sense still remained: hearing. He could hear everything around him, every comment or observation nurses and visitors made. Was this true for Dilys? I asked one of the nurses.

"That's what we're taught," she said.

Hearing is said to be the last of the senses to go. When speech has been lost, either temporarily or permanently, it's easy to forget that a stroke patient may still have excellent hearing. So discussing the patient's condition in front of the patient is unwise: say what you're happy to have heard.

The patient's brain may be damaged, but the mind may still be active. In 'The Diving Bell and the Butterfly', the patient describes how he watched his past life receding, like a sailor watching his home shore gradually disappearing. Although virtually all movement had been lost, he filled the empty hospital hours by taking imaginary journeys to places he remembered, but would never visit again. He prepared imaginary meals, recalling the taste sensations that he would never experience again. He relived old triumphs and disasters from a life he would never live again. Inside a useless body there is often a living, conscious person. That's something never to be forgotten.

I talked to Dilys for a while, telling her about the news from the boys, what her lovely grandchildren were up to, the pleasure of having had Janet to stay, all the little domestic chatter that she must miss. And just occasionally, from that locked-in, motionless form, my hand received the tiniest of squeezes, just to show she was there.

When it was time to go, I asked her about her radio. Now that she was in a room of her own there was no question of it possibly disturbing the other patients. Yes she'd like it on, the squeeze said, and knowing her love of classical music, I left her with Classic FM playing quietly in the background.

The need to see Dr. Phillips was bothering me: this was important for Dilys. Since Sister couldn't help at present, it seemed sensible to try the other route, and approach his secretary for an appointment on his return.

The next afternoon, I thought I'd try to fix the appointment with Dr. Phillips, so after visiting I returned via the main hospital. Although the medical secretary's office was in a strange part of the building, walking through the long, familiar corridors and full wards of that busy world brought back the unhappy feelings I had when Dilys was admitted there, more than two months ago. How much had changed since then.

I knocked and entered. Three girls looked surprised that a visitor had breached what they clearly regarded as a private sanctum. One identified herself as Dr. Phillips's secretary, but couldn't help me.

"I don't know what his movements are," she said. "He'll tell me what he wants to do when he's back from holiday."

Stymied: she certainly wasn't going to enter any appointments in her consultant's diary until he returned. I would have to be patient and wait till he was back.

Meanwhile Dr. Dayala was still in charge.

I asked after Bob. He had been sent home, where social services had arranged for him to have a carer call morning and evening. He'd done well, the nurse said, though he was disappointed that he wasn't able to drive as yet.

Losing the ability to drive is indeed a disappointing blow. But hope should not be abandoned: there are several organisations for disabled drivers. For example, The Disabled Drivers Association is a useful organisation to contact. It aims to promote independence through improved mobility for disabled people and those with disability problems. Among other things, it provides information on the range of vehicles with modified controls that might suit different circumstances.

I had always known that the hospital policy was to return patients to care at home, but as the days and weeks had passed, and Dilys's condition had deteriorated, somehow that likelihood had been pushed to the back of my mind. Bob's going home seemed to be a different matter. Then one morning, sudden shock! One of the nurses reminded me that as Dilys's condition was stabilising, moving her out to free her bed was still a possibility.

"But she'll need a nursing home," the nurse said, "and a good one. She needs total nursing care now, and you certainly won't be able to manage at home."

It took a while to come to terms with this. It meant the end of any thoughts of having Dilys back home. She'd never return to her own house again; we'd never share a life together again; more blows to take. At the same time I felt relieved that the hospital staff were so definite, and that I wasn't being asked to choose. I thought of the toiletting, the hoist, the ripple bed they were using to avoid sores, the turning, the drip feed, the stomach peg. No, being sensible, I'd not be able to manage all those.

I'd have to find a nursing home, and one that had appropriate nursing facilities for her needs, too. That might be difficult. I felt miserable again. I certainly couldn't imagine anywhere that would provide care as good as she was getting in the little hospital.

"When will this happen?" I asked. The nurse read my thoughts.

"Don't do anything yet – we'll give you plenty of notice," she said.

Nevertheless, I felt I had to make plans for the new situation. Somehow, I'd settled too easily into the routine of hospital care for Dilys and my twice daily hospital visiting. When I got home I made a quick list of the nursing homes I knew. Then I remembered a friend of Dilys's who worked for a nursing agency in the area. I rang her, and she called round to see me. Together we went through my list. By the time she left, we'd reduced the list of those that offered the kind of nursing Dilys needed to three. The friend gave her private opinion of all three, based on first hand knowledge. I rang one, to ask if I could visit.

"Sorry, we're closing in a few months, and we're not taking any more patients." Another setback; I decided to leave matters until the hospital told me to prepare for the move. Who could tell now what might be available then?

If it's necessary to find suitable care, get as much information as possible about the placements that are available at the time of deciding. The Social Services Department keeps a list of registered establishments, and this is often a useful start – there may be some in your locality that you weren't aware of. The hospital itself might be able to offer suggestions. You'll want to see the more likely ones for yourself, of course, but try to talk to those who've had first hand experiences there, both as patients and as relatives of patients. Remember too that a change in ownership or management will often have brought a change in the quality of care on offer. In the last resort, however, the placement may have to be decided by what's available at the time, rather than by what's ideal.

The week passed. By now, even the faint squeeze of my hand had disappeared, and there was no response from Dilys at all. I sat in the room by her bedside, watching the slow rise and fall of her chest, listening to Classic FM playing quietly in the background. She looked so clean. She'd always had lovely skin, and even now, in spite of the lack of food, her cheeks, though pale, were almost as full as normal. I kissed her gently on the forehead, and like the sleeping beauty, she suddenly awoke. I saw her eyes open, and saw her yawn. She sat up, smiled, and I heard her say in the voice I knew so well, "Hullo, Huw, haven't I had a lovely sleep."

The moment passed: the wish would never be realised. She was like a living doll; washed, dressed, turned, moved, toiletted by the nurses every day. How she would have hated the indignity of it all if she knew. Or did she know?

When was Dr. Phillips next due to consult at St. Michael's? I asked the nurses, but no one knew. Sister thought he might be coming the following Monday, but wasn't sure. She knew how much I wanted to see him, and promised to find out and arrange an appointment with him. She rang me at home; sorry, she hadn't been able to make contact.

Senior medical staff seemed to be as elusive as the Scarlet Pimpernel, I thought. I decided to have one last go myself, and rang the protective secretary. She was more forthcoming. No, she hadn't heard from him for a day or so either, but she did have him diaried for St. Michael's on Tuesday. I rang Sister with the news.

"You've found out: what a star!" she cried. "I'll put you in for about noon, but the exact time will depend on how the ward round goes of course."

At last; a chance to see the consultant. I wasn't quite sure what I'd gain from the meeting, but I felt that for Dilys's sake as well as mine I needed to get an expert's view of her future, and to ensure that every possible avenue of treatment was being explored. I rang my sons with the news about next Tuesday; Michael said he wanted to be there with me. Good: family support again.

Last week of July and first week of August

The squeeze of the hand had been our only communication. Now that had gone, and when I asked a question, there was no answering squeeze. But in the warm summer weather she was covered by only the lightest of sheets, and I suddenly noticed a very slight movement under the cover. She was moving a toe! I tried again, asking a question.

"If you can hear me Dilys, waggle your toe."

The sheet twitched: no doubt about it, we were in communication again. For a couple of days Dilys was still there, answering 'yes' to questions. In spite of the nourishment she was receiving, the muscles – or rather the ability to move the muscles, had so very nearly gone. The only muscle she could move, out of all the complicated machinery of her body, was just one toe on just one foot. It was still one way traffic, she couldn't express her own wishes and feelings, but at least she was able to give that frail response. Under the sheet, on the bed, inside the nightie, was a living, thinking person, helpless, trapped in her useless body. In spite of the nourishment the deterioration was slowly continuing.

Two days later, even that one movement had gone.

Sometimes the term 'locked-in syndrome' is applied to a variety of conditions where virtually all movement control has been lost, though sometimes eye movement remains. This is often the result of a brainstem stroke. The victim can hear, can think, can feel emotions: the mind is alive, like sunlight playing in a darkened room. Relatives can offer companion-ship, stimulation, and the realisation that this is not a vegetative state. Although the outlook is not good, any slight sign of recovery, especially in the young, is a sign that all hope is not lost.

On Tuesday, Michael arrived early, and we reached the hospital in good time for the appointment with the consultant. Every now and then I peeped outside the door of Dilys's room to see the activity in the ward, the curtains round a bed drawn for privacy, Sister hovering outside with a trolley laden with files, and the little procession then moving on. The clock moved on too, noon, half-past – it was getting on for one o'clock when Sister came in and escorted Michael and me to an interview room.

Dr. Phillips sat behind a desk, Sister on a chair to one side. He looked to be in his late thirties or early forties, I thought, dark suit, tie, brown hair, serious face. He stood to shake hands when we were introduced; a tall man, a good six footer. He began with what I now recognised as standard medical questioning technique – throw the question over to the patient/relative.

"So what would you like to know?"

"First of all, can you confirm what's wrong with Dilys?"

He assured me that he was certain she'd had a brainstem stroke.

"At first, I wanted her to have another scan to make sure," he went on, "but as her illness has progressed, there's really no need for that now. She's not well enough to stand the investigation, anyway."

I felt relieved. Ever since she'd had the traumatic trip to the main hospital for the stomach peg, I'd been secretly dreading another visit there. Moving her out of her comfortable bed, strapping her on to a trolley for the ambulance men, travelling through the little lanes picking up other patients while she lay in the back of the vehicle, waiting for the appointment, waiting again for an ambulance for the return journey – what an ordeal for her. Thank goodness that wouldn't be necessary.

Dr. Phillips had obviously been primed about our main concerns. He came straight to the issue of food or water.

"One of the effects of her stroke is that she's quite unable to swallow. Dr. Dayala's decision on the stomach peg was absolutely right," he went on. "If I'd been here when the feeding question arose I'd have made exactly the same decision."

For a moment I sensed the leader backing his staff, right or wrong, but then dismissed the thought. He seemed too straightforward.

I reached into my pocket. "I've brought statements from all the family, testifying to Dilys's wishes if she were ever in a situation like this. Would you like to see them?"

He waved the papers aside. "No point," he said. "And by the way, there's no point in having a neurologist's opinion, either."

A double whammy. I didn't feel strong enough to challenge either point.

"So how do you see her chances of recovery and of coming home?" I asked.

He looked directly at me. "Recovery from a stroke usually starts within six weeks, though there are cases of a longer delay."

This is the point at which recovery starts and the patient begins to regain lost functions. Thereafter, the chances of recovery, though still present, are diminished. Recovery from a major stroke is a long term process, and once it starts, patients can continue to improve gradually for a year or more.

I didn't need to calculate how long it was since Dilys started to feel ill – between nine and 10 weeks.

I interpreted his answer. "Does that mean virtually no chance?" I asked.

He spoke more gently. "I'm afraid so."

I pressed him further. "So how long do you think Dilys has got?"

At first he gave the stock answer. "No one can predict that," he said. But then he looked straight at me again, pausing as if summing up whether I could accept bad news, before continuing, "I would say, for someone in Dilys's condition, about a month, unless she gets an infection."

At last I had something more definite to go on. The months that the senior Sister had mentioned were now reduced to one. Dilys only had to endure a few more weeks before she could rest for ever. I took out my handkerchief to wipe my eyes. I felt Michael's arm around my shoulders as I heard Dr. Phillips's voice, coming as if from a distance.

"I don't think she'd be here now were it not for the superb nursing care she's getting."

That comment was clearly one for Sister, as much as me. But I did feel strong enough to want to say how much I appreciated what the nurses were doing.

"Indeed so," I said. "The whole family will endorse that."

I asked about the next step.

"This is only a short stay hospital," he said, "and we do transfer patients out when they are ready."

"So should I be looking for a nursing home?"

"Not immediately; leave it for a fortnight or so."

I thanked him for his time, and we left to see Dilys before going for lunch. As we passed the nursing station, Sister caught my arm.

"Don't worry about a nursing home," she whispered. "I'll not want to let her go from here."

I felt a great relief. Sister had removed one worry. At least poor Dilys would be well nursed for her last days.

All strokes are different: not all strokes are life threatening, not all strokes involve the same loss of functions. Even after severe brainstem strokes, some patients live for years, and a few patients do make some recovery. What all stroke victims need and deserve is the best of nursing care and the best of support and encouragement. The better these are, the better the chances of recovery.

I continued talking to Dilys when I visited. She'd perhaps enjoy hearing the news, the talk, the gossip about the familiar life she knew. She had all the rest of the long nights to make her peace with the world she was leaving. One way conversations with no response at all were strange, but I prepared a list of topics before leaving to visit each day, so that I wouldn't dry up, with nothing to say. And I'd see that her radio continued playing the music from her favourite programme, Classic FM.

Preparing what a stroke patient – any patient – might like to hear from you is quite a useful approach to hospital visiting. If you're going to spend, as I did, a couple of hours each morning and again each afternoon as sole visitor in the ward, it becomes important. Your patient will be interested in friends, hobbies, local gossip, news, relatives – so many things. It's useful to write the list of topics on a card to take with you.

Later in the week I mentioned Dilys's future to one of the nurses. She confirmed what Sister had said.

"She definitely won't be going home. She needs total nursing."

No doubt: that was final. That evening I looked in the spare bedroom. The wheelchair I'd fetched in May, when the district nurse felt it would help her mobility, stood in the corner. I wouldn't need it now. Next morning, before visiting, I loaded it into the car and returned it to the central store. I felt a pang to see it go: with it went another hope.

Second week of August

A big family weekend: everybody seemed to come. Our older son and family stayed with me for three nights, our Australian son-in-law happened to be working in the UK for a brief period, and he arrived, as did our younger son. Everyone visited Dilys. I'd warned them beforehand that they shouldn't expect any response from her now: for the last few days she had sunk into a comatose state.

I prepared the accommodation. The two little grandsons liked the attic room; they enjoy being independent, quite cut off from the grown-ups, who all sleep on the bungalow's ground floor. We're close to the shore, and the boys love coming to visit.

"Come and play skip-stones, Taid," they commanded immediately, calling me by the Welsh name for grandfather.

I forgot everything else, gave priority to the grandchildren, and went with them to the water's edge. The younger lad managed 10 skips: hadn't he improved since last time! I was back in the normal world again, a world of family outings and games with grandchildren.

It's sometimes a temptation to behave like a hermit and withdraw to the equivalent of a personal cell while the all-consuming stroke occupies your thoughts. This can be a mistake. An occasional escape to normality is beneficial in so many ways, and returning to the life of the family is a particularly encouraging experience.

I suddenly realised I wasn't thinking of Dilys, and hadn't thought of her since the family had arrived. Is this good, I wondered? And I didn't have to bother about meals, since our daughter-in-law took over the cooking for all of us. She even washed and tumble-dried their sheets and towels on the morning they left. What a great character!

If people ask about coming to stay (and some do, often thinking you would be glad of company) say quite openly that you can't do meals for them, leaving them to sort out how they'll manage. And it's no offence to ask whether they'd be willing to bring sleeping bags, to save changing beds and sheets. There is enough to worry about without thinking of feeding visitors and managing extra chores. If they suggest eating out, or offer to cook, and to do the washing, hold them to it.

If the thought of visitors really worries you, don't hesitate to say that it's a busy time, and you'd prefer to see them later on.

Relatives, and friends who you know will help are different, of course.

On the other hand, you may prefer to have jobs to do while others do the hospital visiting. Absorption in routine tasks may take the mind off more worrying matters.

Dilys enjoyed a lovely relationship with the two boys, and they in turn were very fond of their grandmother, or Nain, as they called her. Their parents had discussed carefully whether the boys should see their grandmother in her changed state. Would it upset them? Would it be more worrying if they didn't see her? They decided that their father would take them to the hospital on his own. The hospital itself would be a strange experience for them. Then if the boys were able to handle that, and wanted to see Dilys, he would take them in to see her. He talked over with them what to expect.

Whether to take children to see stroke patients depends on many things. The age of the child is one, the relationship with the patient is another. The decision rests with the parents, who know the children best. The hospital, too, may have a view on this, though the presence of children is usually a cheering glimpse of normality for staff and patients alike.

What is clear is that taking children to see stroke patients does need preparation. The sight of a familiar, well loved member of the family in a very different state from usual, perhaps unable to talk to them, unable to hug them, perhaps looking helpless, is upsetting. If it's unexpected, it can be unnecessarily traumatic. So a little explanation beforehand of what to expect, and a discussion of the questions that children usually raise is well worthwhile.

The boys, aged six and eight, had been prepared for the quiet of the hospital, the very old people lying in beds, or trying to use zimmers, and the uniformed nurses. They were still overawed by the reality: this was a new, strange experience. They weren't sure now that they wanted to venture further, and go in to their Nain's room. But then Sister appeared on the scene.

"What lovely boys," she exclaimed, "what are your names?" The familiar question eased the uncertainty, and as they started to chat, the atmosphere became less strange, and they relaxed. The passing nurses smiled warmly at the little visitors; not many children came to this hospital.

"Come and see your Nain for a minute," Sister said, and taking their hands, walked with them into Dilys's room, where she left them with their father. There was no point in a long visit, and shortly afterwards, their father brought them out again. Later, we talked over the visit with them. They wanted to have the feeding machine explained, and to know why Dilys couldn't eat.

Discussion afterwards is as important as preparation beforehand. Children can have odd fantasies and worries about new experiences, perhaps particularly about illness and hospitals, and they need the chance to bring them out and to have any irrational worries dispelled. Questions must be answered honestly.

"Wasn't Nain quiet," the younger one said, remembering the lively, outgoing grandmother she had been. "Will she always be like this now?" The innocent question hurt.

"Probably," I said quietly.

Our son-in-law came late on Saturday, and visited Dilys on the Sunday morning. I kept our daughter and family well posted with news of Dilys; New Zealand was very far away, and I guessed they worried more than the rest of the family. I expected the son-in-law had been briefed to check that I hadn't been playing down her condition, and to report how I was managing, too. They needn't have worried about me, but I knew they did.

With so many visitors for Dilys it was an opportunity to call in to see Bob. I'd heard from friends that he'd settled well. "But he can be demanding," one said, "not like Bob at all. He's more irritable than I remember. I suspect he's feeling angry at what's happened and taking it out on us," she said understandingly.

Stroke patients can feel angry. 'Why has this happened to me?' they ask themselves. 'It's unfair,' they cry, seeing older friends with all their abilities still intact. And unfairness makes any one of us angry. Our tolerance is often difficult, but necessary.

I found Bob feeling more positive than I had been led to believe. The carers were coming as arranged, he was beginning to return to some of his old interests, and he'd had some useful advice over the financial support available.

The social worker is a key person in this phase of the recovery programme. The role is centrally concerned with providing carers and liaising with the medical services. But don't forget to ask also about the various allowances that individuals with loss of functions are entitled to receive. There are extra expenses – perhaps taxis to and from medical appointments for example – and additional funds are important.

Our younger son came and visited Dilys as arranged on Sunday afternoon, and by the evening everyone had gone. I had hoped that somehow the family visitors might have stirred some response from Dilys. But no one, not even her grandchildren, evoked any change in the motionless form in the empty room. Did she know they had been there, had she tried to open an eye, to lift a hand, to raise a smile? Yes, she did know, and she'd tried: I felt certain of that. But inside that useless prison of a body, how did she feel when she couldn't react, couldn't reach out to them, no matter how hard she tried? Who knows?

The weekend had passed, the family had gone, and the regular pattern of hospital visits, hospital washing, and the chores of cooking and cleaning returned. The familiar routine was punctuated by occasional notes in the empty calendar. Some were practical issues; when the consultant might be available; reminders to buy more essentials for Dilys – soap, or scent, or batteries for her bedside radio. Others were events to look forward to; the once or twice every week when neighbours and friends took turns to invite me out to dinner. I felt privileged to enjoy such kindness, the balm of humanity providing a balance to the uncaring, unfair brutality of Dilys's stroke.

As I drove through the town to the hospital I noticed how busy the town was; visitors on holiday by the water, local children playing their holidays away. August: school holidays of course. August: something else nagged away, an uneasy itch that asked to be noticed. I scratched. What was it? At last I hit it: relief. Of course, August: at the end of the week it would be our wedding anniversary!

I suddenly felt depressed. This would be our last anniversary, no doubt about it. How could I look forward to our wedding anniversary, knowing that it would be the last? This would be the end of the sequence, our fifty-third and our final one. I couldn't celebrate it under these circumstances. Or could I? Dilys would like there to be a celebration, of that I was sure. But what sort of celebration, and in what way?

If Dilys and I couldn't enjoy our anniversary together, at least I ought to mark it in some way. It wasn't the sort of occasion to invite friends and family; that would be bizarre. But the hospital staff; they deserved a big 'thank you' for looking after her on her wedding anniversary. I went to the best chocolate shop in town and bought the biggest box of chocolates there.

"Enjoy these," I said to Sister. "It's our wedding anniversary, and we'd like you and your colleagues to celebrate it for us."

Because someone is the victim of a stroke, whether in hospital or at home, celebrations should not be forgotten. Indeed they are in many ways more important still. Remembering birthdays, anniversaries, special occasions of any sort – this helps the patient to feel part of everyday living, rather than feeling isolated and cut off.

In the room Dilys was lying as quietly as ever. When I looked carefully I could see the feeding machine pulsing the drops of life sustaining fluid and the gentle rise and fall of her chest. There was no other sign of life. I sat down in my usual chair, held her hand, and thought of anniversaries past. I let my mind pour out the memories, and I reminded her of that first year, living in our little rented flat on the South Downs, both of us teaching, when we two young marrieds in our early twenties walked across the Surrey weald to the White Hart in Bletchingley. I remembered the bottle of wine I ordered with the meal – a Chateauneuf du Pape. Why did that detail stay with me, I wondered. For a present I'd bought her a dressing table set, but she told me she'd never want presents, just the memory of happy days. After that I'd always bought flowers; those she loved and would always accept, but she didn't want our money spent on mementoes for herself. She was always a practical girl, a great household manager. I reminded her of that, too, hoping for a sign, a pressure of the hand, the twitch of a smile, any sign of acknowledgement. Nothing.

I reminded her of a later anniversary, one which had fallen on a weekend. I'd brought a surprise picnic basket full of delicacies. I smiled as I recalled them: smoked salmon, cheese, baguettes, grapes, melon and a bottle of champagne. We'd driven to Berkshire, and we'd picnicked where I'd lived as an adolescent. Dilys and I were working in Southampton on that occasion, and we'd just bought our first car, a little Austin A30. Must have been our fifth or sixth anniversary. She'd know which one it was. I wondered sadly if she was trying to tell me, I wondered what thoughts were playing inside that unreachable isolation.

Naturally I remembered the twenty-fifth very clearly. I was working in western Canada, and we spent the anniversary walking in the Rockies, in the Waterston-Glacier National Park. I remembered the very friendly waitress at the restaurant. "You two look happy," she said. We told her why, and she produced a small cake from the kitchen, topped with a candle. Funny the little events that stay in memory. Optimistically, we said we'd go back there for our fiftieth, but of course we didn't.

We'd made the fiftieth something special. Over 30 family members had travelled to our wedding lunch and evening buffet. Our New Zealand family – daughter, son-in-law and all their children – had come over, and we'd had some lovely photographs. It hadn't been as perfect as we'd hoped – there'd been a bit of an argument beforehand with the hotel, but what mattered was that she and I had stood together over it, and I reminded her of that, too. The family gathering had proved to be a very happy occasion, and that was the most important memory. I told her how we were celebrating this anniversary. How I hoped she heard me.

Once again, talk about what's happening. Even patients who are apparently in a completely unresponsive state may well be able to hear you. You may never know how much comfort your talking will give; just assume that it's reaching an active mind, stimulating shared memories, enriching the drabness of totally inactive days.

Photographs! When our older son had last visited he'd said how bare the room was. The fiftieth anniversary provided the answer. Among the photographs, one was Dilys's favourite, a shot of the two of us, surrounded by our three children, their partners, and the seven grandchildren. Everyone was smiling happily. I'll bring that in to the hospital, I decided, and put it up above her bed, as a memory of happy days. When I tell her, she'll be pleased. The next day I pinned the photograph up, and I smiled as I told her.

"What a happy photograph," the nurse said, when she looked in.

"I recognise your daughter and the two sons from their visits. When was it taken?"

I told her it was our fiftieth wedding anniversary, and showed her which grandchildren belonged to which family.

"We've been very lucky," I added. "It's been 53 years, and though it's all ending now, what great years they've been." I hoped Dilys had heard that. I felt the lump in my throat.

"I'm so glad you can look at things like that," the nurse said. "It makes all the difference." As she went out of the room, she closed the door behind her, leaving the two of us alone.

Third week of August

The lovely summer continued. My routine was fully established now; pack a small lunch, drive to the hospital, not forgetting the clean nightie, which I'd washed by hand, greet the nursing staff, ask how the night had gone, and then go straight to Dilys. The room would be as immaculate as ever, the radio playing Classic FM, and Dilys sleeping; changed, washed and still. The room was not quite as still as it seemed at first. There was the regular movement in the ripple bed, the steady drip of the feeding bottle on its stand, the second hand circling the face of the wall clock, and the gentle rise and fall of Dilys's breathing. Not still, but peaceful. I always had an odd feeling on entering; it was hard to believe that dying could be so restful.

I'd then kiss Dilys, and start to talk to her. I'd gently stroke her arm, hoping that she could feel the touch, though not knowing, since loss of feeling might well be another effect of the stroke.

After a couple of hours of sitting, chatting, listening to the music, it was time for lunch. The little hospital lay on the outskirts of a small market town, and I knew that there was a new nature reserve close by. Each lunchtime, in what seemed that summer's permanent sunshine, I walked through the reserve entrance, past the wooden sculptures, along the path beside the river, until the path crossed the bridge and I reached my favourite seat. The bright green of the young May leaves had now started to dull into the full flush of summer maturity, the excited birdsong in the woodland had begun to quieten: the year was moving on. I ate my lunch and walked back to the hospital.

After lunch the nurses always came to change Dilys, and I'd leave the room while they saw to her. They usually altered her position, and so afterwards I'd move the chair to the other side of the bed to talk to her. The afternoon was a repeat of the morning; I'd tell Dilys about the lunchtime walk, the people I'd seen, how her beloved garden was looking, whether I'd bought her any soap or scent: all trivialities, but which nevertheless kept her in touch with the life she was leaving. Sometimes a hospital visitor, someone who had volunteered to make regular visits to the patients, would look in and have a chat with me.

The next room was occupied by another lady of about the same age as Dilys. She too had suffered a stroke, and like Dilys, was bedridden and couldn't speak. She could smile, and I made it a point to stop outside the door and say hello from the open doorway.

I'd have a word with the nurses and the domestic staff, too, and gradually heard about their families, their holidays, their pattern of duties. I felt I was now a member of the hospital community, and understood more easily the wonderful service they provided.

It's obvious that getting on good terms with the hospital staff makes life more pleasant for everyone. This can sometimes be forgotten, when you have the best interests of a stroke victim at heart, and are under pressure and stress yourself. Of course the whistle has to be blown over slovenly practices. But before criticising, it's worth pausing to ask yourself whether you would improve on the 24/7 care that your relative is receiving from the hospital staff.

During the week the nutrition drip was reduced from 75mls to 50mls. I assumed that as Dilys was completely inactive she needed less. Then a couple of days later her nurse stopped me as I entered the room. She told me that Dilys was now completely comatose. Her eyes had been opening occasionally when they changed her in the mornings, but even that had now stopped, and apart from the breathing, she was lifeless. They had therefore taken the feeding drip away and put her on water only. I looked at the drip. The clear, colourless liquid told its own story. I felt a sickness at the bottom of my stomach. The roller coaster was beginning what would be its last run downhill.

I rang the children to tell them. Their reaction was relief, followed by immediate sympathy for me.

Yet again, children can play such an important role in supporting relatives of stroke victims. This can't be overstressed.

"We'll come up to see you," both boys said.

"I'll get a flight at once," Janet said

"No," I said, feeling an immediate surge of gratitude for their reaction, "there's no immediate need to come. I'll let you know how things go."

It was a blow, a sickening blow, none the easier for having been expected. Yet for all of us, depression was shot through with glimpses of relief.

It was John's turn to send me a book.

"I found this helpful, Dad," said the note accompanying it. I looked at the title: 'A Good Death'.

The book was written by a GP. She had met many relatives of the dying who were anxious or worried about the impending death, often the first death at which they had been present. What happened? Did they need to do anything in preparation? Did they need to do anything afterwards? The book's purpose was to take people who might be troubled, worried, uncertain, through the mystery of death. It described in simple, reassuring words, the physical process of dying, and described common reactions to loss. It also mentioned the formalities involved, the official steps that had to be taken. Like 'The Diving Bell and the Butterfly' it provided help at a difficult time.

Fortunately, most stroke victims recover, but nevertheless death is always a possibility, difficult to face. If recovery is unlikely, then it is really important to be ready to come to terms with the emotional and practical realities. There are other publications beside the one mentioned which give good advice on coping, and a couple of helpful ones are given in the list of useful sources of information. Several organisations that have to be contacted after death has occurred, such as the Registry of Births and Deaths and the Probate Office, also provide helpful pamphlets. But some individuals have little idea of the procedures to be followed, and may worry beforehand about what to do. Often the best preparation is to talk with an understanding friend who has had to cope with a recent bereavement, and who can reassure you over the help you will receive.

Bob had by now been discharged and had gone home. A couple of years ago he'd moved from his semi-bungalow and was living on his own in a small flat in sheltered accommodation with a warden on site. At 85, that seemed entirely sensible. The flat was overfull: a large settee and a couple of armchairs occupied most of the floor space, books filled the long shelves on two walls and dribbled out over the two tables and on to the floor.

His speech, though still slurred, had begun to improve and he was able to move about with the aid of a stick. There was hope that his mobility would improve still further. Like so many stroke victims, he was definitely on the road to recovery, another success for the rehabilitation team. Good for him, I thought.

I couldn't help reflecting about the different outcomes of the strokes that Bob and Dilys had suffered. There was Bob, recovering well, and here was Dilys...

For the rest of the week Dilys lay motionless. Occasionally she would be troubled by catarrh in her throat, which of course she couldn't swallow, and a nurse would come and use a suction tube to remove it.

Towards the end of the week I noticed a change. Dilys was breathing more rapidly, and her skin looked dry. Her mouth was slightly open; she clearly wasn't well. I saw the nurse.

"Yes, she has a little infection," she said.

"Are you giving her anything for it?" I asked.

The nurse looked at me. "Mild painkillers in her drip," she said. "But if you want her to have antibiotics I'll tell the doctor."

My mind flashed back to our discussions with the doctors a few weeks ago. In theory, it seemed so much kinder to let a dying patient – for that was what Dilys now was – pass away untreated. The alternative, to try to help her recover, meant that with her weakened body she'd only suffer the same trauma over and over again, until eventually she became too weak to recover.

In practice, face to face with the sick, struggling patient, theory is threatened by loving sympathy. A short course of antibiotics would ease her immediate suffering, and she'd be back to her previous peaceful state. Should she be treated? Nobody, let alone a loved and loving partner, should be allowed to suffer unnecessarily. I looked at Dilys, pale and breathing rapidly;

for a moment I weakened. The nurse waited. What should I say?

I hesitated. Then I suddenly found a guiding principle. What would Dilys have wanted? And I knew very well what she would have wanted. I turned away from the nurse, biting my lip.

"Just carry on with the painkillers," I said.

No one can ever forecast every eventuality. But it does help to try to prepare for difficult decisions that might have to be faced, even though the reality may be hard to imagine beforehand. The medical personnel will have seen others in similar situations, and will know what choice points are likely to occur, so they can be helpful in alerting you to the possibilities you might have to face. And talk about the alternatives with the family beforehand.

Nothing can leave more bitterness than divisions within a family over the course of care for a relative. Try very hard to reach a united view. The death of a relative is difficult enough to suffer, without having to deal with recriminations from within the family afterwards. Early discussions make it easier to reach an agreed course of action: the pressure of having to take a quick decision which has not been previously agreed within the family can lead to rifts which are difficult to heal.

Her illness continued, no worse, but no better. To keep a lay-man's eye on her condition I counted her rate of breathing, timing the rise and fall of her chest against the second hand on my watch. Thirty-five, thirty-six per minute, not very good. Two days later the rate started to fall, and by the end of the week it was down to the low twenties, and she looked more as she was at the start of the week.

"Yes, she's better," the nurse said. "She must have a tough constitution."

Last week of August

Dilys was now completely comatose, sleeping undisturbed, day and night. My lovely, lively life's companion was no longer with me. I lived in a strange, detached world, continuing to visit, continuing to talk to her, continuing to ensure that her music was playing gently from the radio beside her bed. It all seemed unreal, dream-like. Then Sister stopped me as I came in one morning.

"Ah, Mr Watkins! Now you handed in Dilys's kidney donor card when she was admitted, I think."

I'd forgotten about that: it seemed such a long time since Dilys had arrived at the hospital, talking a little, smiling, waving to the other patients. I remembered the card. What was coming, I wondered, remembering her wishes over the use of her body for others. Sister continued.

"The transplant nurse is coming in this afternoon to talk to the nurses about tissue donation, and I thought you might like to meet her and have a word with her. About four o'clock, if that's convenient."

It was convenient, and if it wasn't I'd have made it so. Why did she want to see me?

A tall lady, not in nurse's uniform, came to Sister's desk shortly after four o'clock. She introduced herself as Julia, the transplant nurse, and took me down the corridor, past Dilys's room, to the guest room, used for overnight stays. We settled into comfortable armchairs.

Julia was a very pleasant person, in her thirties, I thought, and with a gentle, approachable manner. She began by asking about my background, where I was from, where I'd worked, and so on. I recognised the process of talking about familiarities, in order to put me at my ease, and I felt very comfortable, sitting there in the armchair, describing our family and our life to this interested listener.

Then Julia turned to the point of the meeting. Would I be able to reassure her that Dilys definitely wanted her body to be used in this way?

"Definitely," I replied confidently, remembering Dilys's strong views on being useful to others.

That clearly pleased Julia, who then explained, as Sister had done previously, that there were developments in tissue donation: things had moved on, and the kidney donor card that Dilys carried had been superseded. There was now an Organ Donor Register, a national organisation dealing not only with kidneys but with other tissues that could be used to help ill patients.

"In any case," Julia went on, "kidney donation would be inappropriate for Dilys. It's used only for live, healthy kidneys, like those from fit patients on life support machines after car accidents."

I absorbed this: the implication being that poor Dilys's

kidneys might not have been suitable after her prolonged period of illness.

"But other tissues could perhaps be used," Julia went on. She listed body parts that could be donated for helping other people in need. I knew that healthy hearts could be donated. But in addition, skin could be taken for skin grafts; eyes for transplanting; bone, too. I was taken aback at the several different body parts that could be used. These would have to be taken immediately after death, and I would need to complete a donor form for this to happen. She handed me a form and an information leaflet.

Immediately after death... that phrase made me pause. It might be that one of her children couldn't be with her when she died, and would arrive, wanting to see her one last time. But the pathologists would be at work on the body immediately after death. What condition would the body be in? I put that difficulty to Julia.

She was clearly used to the question.

"That wouldn't be a problem," Julia said. "She'd be dressed normally, there'd be prostheses in the eyes, the lids would be closed... really no one would know the difference."

Suddenly my self-composure began to melt like snow under the sun. Here I was, calmly discussing what bits to cut out of a dead body and how to replace them artificially. This was ghoulish. The decision to offer to donate organs had seemed so right all those years ago, when death was something a long

way away. To help others to live was a good action; its consequences lay far off, in a distant future. That future was suddenly the here and now; it had to be faced. Worse, much worse,
this talk of body parts was no longer an impersonal, abstract
discussion about a lifeless body. It was about my lovely Dilys,
while she lay, living and breathing, just two doors away,
unable to contribute; I was talking about doing this to her
while she lay ill and helpless. I felt horrible. The relaxed,
unemotional atmosphere suddenly changed, and my eyes
filled with tears, the first time for months.

As a relative, the key point is to be prepared for this as far as this is possible. It's easy to take a decision, forget about it, and years later suddenly face unexpected and upsetting realities; no one wants to think regularly about death. But after a serious stroke, when the patient perhaps
cannot communicate, the possibility of tissue donation may arise. Don't
let this happen at a difficult time: if possible, read about the procedures,
think about the questions you want to ask, and be ready to ask them.
Talk to those who are familiar with the procedures before the moment
of decision arrives.

Julia was shocked. "I'll get a cup of tea," she said, and shot out
of the room, returning shortly, when I apologised for my lack
of control. Sister came in with tea and biscuits. Julia then
apologised for upsetting me.

"Are you sure you want to go on with this?" she asked. "Why
don't you take a little time to think about it, and let me know
later."

"No," I said. The principle that had previously guided me – and the children – was the right one to follow. It was what Dilys would have wanted.

"We'll go ahead."

There is no doubt that some people are unable to consider tissue donation, perhaps on religious, or moral or other grounds. That view is entirely proper, and must be respected. But helping the living by tissue donation after death is an action that appeals to many of us, and if you feel this way, make your wishes known by completing the appropriate form, and placing a copy where it can be easily found.

The end of the week came, and with it another shock, another dive on the roller coaster. On the Friday, the nurse caught me in the corridor as I walked towards Dilys's room.

"We saw signs of returning consciousness this morning. When we changed her, her eyes followed us around the room, and she seemed to respond to our voices."

A flash of hope. An incredible, unbelievable recovery? In spite of Dr. Phillips? The nurse read my expression.

"People with serious strokes do sometimes get short periods of surfacing from coma, usually short periods only." Short period only... no hope then.

"But the doctor may want to restart feeding," she went on.

Restart feeding! To what purpose, I thought, if this is a

momentary phase. This was dragging Dilys out of a peaceful sea, and beaching her briefly on the stony shore of life before the tide carried her out again.

"We'll do nothing over the weekend," she said. "We'll discuss it with the doctor on Monday."

I went in to see Dilys, my feelings in a turmoil. What was the point of this cat and mouse game with life? If there was any chance of a recovery, that would be a different matter.

Dilys was sleeping and breathing peacefully. I couldn't evoke any response, either by touching, or talking. Into my mind came a couplet that I remembered from a school magazine, written by a wartime refugee from Hitler's Germany.

When the nights are wet with weeping
And the days are dry with doubt.

The weeping didn't describe my present situation, but the deep uncertainties, the stresses conveyed by the words certainly did.

Perhaps more than any other illness, a stroke can evoke alternating periods of hope aroused and hope dashed. A relative often feels helpless, but never forget that regular visiting helps; just sitting beside the bed, just holding hands, just talking gently – this gives the feeling of support that encourages the patient, and gives point to your own place in the treatment process. You can help by merely being there.

Always be prepared for the times when emotions fluctuate between depression and hope. Knowing that the illness will lead to these won't stop them happening of course, but it will help you meet them when they arrive.

Both sons rang. I'd almost forgotten that it was my birthday that weekend.

Both had decided to come to see us, and take me out for a meal. After they'd visited Dilys we ate at a table we'd booked at a local pub, one we'd not patronised before. The different surroundings, the news of my grandsons, the talk about developments at their work all helped to bring me back to the real world.

"We're thinking of cancelling our holidays," they told me. They'd arranged a joint family camping holiday for the first week of September, just before school started. I thought of the grandsons.

"You mustn't," I said. I knew how disappointed the little boys would be.

Moreover they would all be in this country, just as accessible by phone as if they were at home. Once again I thought of Dilys.

"Your Mum would want you to go, I'm sure of that," I said. And my mind reverted to the drama being played out in the hospital.

First fortnight of September

During the weekend, Dilys had been kept on water only. Monday morning came, and with it, a feeling of approaching unhappiness. Whatever was decided, whether to return Dilys to feeding, or whether to leave her on the finality of water, I would feel a blow. I saw Dr. Dayala disappearing into her office, followed by two or three nurses. This would be the case conference, no doubt. Briefly, I wondered whether the partner of the patient might have been allowed to participate. Perhaps not, I thought: they knew my position very well. So I sat by the bedside, talking to Dilys, who was as unresponsive as ever, while in the background, Classic FM played quietly.

During that long summer I grew to know the Classic FM programmes well. I played the station on the car radio when I drove to and from the hospital, and I made sure that it was playing when I left Dilys at the end of each afternoon's visit. She had often put it on at home, and if, as I hoped, she could hear, she would enjoy it even now.

A piece of music, like a particular smell, can often evoke a whole flood of memories. When I hear a tenor singing 'The Lark in the Clear Air', I'm back in the 1950s, it's a sunny Spring day and I'm walking with Dilys on the South Downs. I can feel the breeze on my cheeks, the pull of the pack on my back and the bounce of the sheep cropped turf under my feet.

Classic FM often played a programme of listeners' favourites, and one particular piece featured regularly, a new piece to me,

'The Ashokan Farewell'. Ashokan was a camp in the Catskill mountains, in New England, where the piece was composed. It was a particularly haunting piece of music, introduced by a plaintive violin, the melody then picked up and carried on by the other instruments, sad yet soothing. I wondered if the title, with its note of a 'goodbye' perhaps struck an additional chord with me, as I sat by the bedside, watching Dilys gradually fade. When I heard it at home it took me straight to the little room with its vase of flowers on the windowsill, the drip of the feeding bottle and Dilys lying motionless under the sheet.

The nurse came in at lunchtime, case conference over. She saw the unspoken question in my expression.

"We decided to keep Dilys on water only."

Once again I felt that mixture of emotions. Once again I had to face the fact that I would soon lose Dilys; yet once again I felt relieved that the right decision, in my view, had been taken.

I apologised to the nurse for having been upset when she'd raised the possibility of restarting feeding.

"You'd be a hard man if you hadn't been," she said.

For the small minority of stroke victims who are unable to ingest food normally, are totally incapacitated and in a coma, decisions about feeding have to be faced. There is no straightforward answer. A living will, as mentioned earlier, is helpful in interpreting the patient's wishes. Decisions, either way, are undoubtedly easier when the patient's known views, the relatives' beliefs and the attitude of the medical staff are all in harmony.

At the time of writing, a draft bill is being prepared for Parliament to debate.

The glorious summer weather got hotter, and I asked for a fan for Dilys's room, which wasn't air conditioned. The temperature rose still higher, and I noticed that the fan had to be shared with other rooms. So I brought in a fan of my own.

Hospitals may not be able to provide everything for the patient's comfort. If there's something which would improve matters, ask the staff for it. It may not be possible to meet an unusual request, so be prepared to help yourself.

I noticed that she had developed small pressure sores on her ears, from lying on the pillow.

When the nurse treated them, she reassured me that these were the only ones.

"The usual places are the heels and the back," she said, "but Dilys is quite clear." It was the ripple bed, apparently which was so valuable in preventing them. And I could see that Dilys was being turned and changed regularly. She continued to look very comfortable, peaceful and pain free.

Her appearance was changing gradually now. She was distinctly paler, though her cheeks still had a fullness which, when I saw her, always made me think for a moment that she was sleeping, and might so easily wake. But by the end of the second week her mouth was hanging open, whereas previously it had always been shut, apart from when she was ill.

"It's a sign of increasing weakness," the nurses said.

Against this steady change in Dilys's condition, my routine continued as before. Each morning I arrived at the hospital, getting cheery greetings from the Sister, the nurses and ward staff. Each morning I'd ask how the night had been, and then talk to Dilys, tell her the snippets of news of family and local gossip, and give her the love sent by relatives and friends. (The cards at home had soon covered all the places used for Christmas cards, and were now spilling over into the kitchen.)

Cards are a comfort, and much less intrusive than phone calls. Many cards are usually sent to the stroke victim in the hospital ward, but the relatives shouldn't be forgotten. Friends and family sometimes think that it's better not to intrude on private distress, but for you, the relative, to know that you are in their thoughts, is helpful. The children often sent me a card, as well as phoning: it's an easy act to choose an interesting or peaceful picture and add a couple of words. But it can mean a lot.

I'd occasionally pause and listen to the radio music with her, and then at lunch it would be time to walk off to the nature reserve, sit quietly with my sandwiches, listen to the calm sound of the little river, and walk back. More chatting after lunch, until the nurses came in for one of Dilys's regular changes of clothes and position, when I went out to say hello to some of the other patients.

One evening I gave Bob a ring; I didn't feel like visiting him. He was getting on quite well, he told me, but finding space in the flat, or lack of it, a bit of a problem. I thought of the zimmer and stick that he'd acquired and would have to accommodate.

"I had a bit of a fright yesterday," he said. "I tripped over the edge of a rug and nearly fell. So I've thrown the rug out."

I thought of the clutter on the floor of Bob's flat, and wasn't surprised.

"Quite right," I said, "and get rid of everything else on the floor too. It's a danger, and you can't pick the stuff up anyway."

Bob chuckled: I could imagine his shamefaced grin, and wondered if he'd do anything about his beloved books.

It's just common sense to remove anything that might be a hazard. It's so easy to promise to do it, but equally easy to omit to do so, particularly if the rug, or piece of furniture, is an old friend. And don't forget about always parking the zimmer or wheelchair in a safe and regular place, especially if vision has been affected. Bob did trip again over the corner of his zimmer. It would have been an irony indeed if he'd been injured by a piece of equipment designed to help.

I'd become quite friendly with the husband of the lady in the room next to Dilys. He and his wife had just moved into new accommodation, a small convenient flat, close to their daughter, a week before she'd had her stroke. He was adjusting to new surroundings, as well as his wife's illness. By now, the smile she used to give me when I waved no longer appeared, and, like Dilys, she lay there, eyes closed, quiet and still. One morning he and his adult children were gathered round her bedside. Today, the bed was empty, the room deserted.

The nurses finished in Dilys's room, so it was back to the bedside for more talk and music until it was time to pick up the washing and drive home to prepare a meal.

Like my own routine, the hospital routine continued too. Nurses went off on their family summer holidays and returned with stories of distant shores; patients were discharged, and their beds soon filled with new arrivals. Life continued.

We had always enjoyed hill-walking, and although we no longer reached the high tops, we still enjoyed a weekend ramble. Since Dilys's illness, I'd had no time for that. Other interests continued. The garden was a great source of pleasure, and during the long evenings of that lovely summer I found calm in my vegetable plot. The flowerbeds and pots had always been Dilys's hobby, and I approached these not with calmness, but with a fierce pleasure, determined to keep them in good shape for her sake, tending them with care, determined that even though Dilys was fading, her plants would continue to bloom defiantly.

Another of our hobbies was contract bridge, a game that has to be played in pairs. Without Dilys, I had no partner, but friends at the bridge club were very thoughtful and often rang up to say that someone was without a partner that evening for various reasons, and to ask whether I'd like to play. I had no hesitation – I always seized the opportunity. There was no point in languishing at home when there was the chance of a social evening to give a contrast to a life of hospital visits. But many evenings no one was free, and I stayed at home.

Then one day the chairman of the club had a brief word with me. A new lady had asked if there was any chance of playing in the club. Of course she'd want a regular partner. He was hesitant about approaching me, but would I like to think about it.

I did. Dilys had been my regular bridge partner since I started playing, nearly 20 years ago. Before that she'd played regularly with someone else; that hadn't worried me. We'd occasionally played with other partners when one of us had been unwell; again, no problems. I felt she would have wanted me to go ahead and play with a regular partner. But on this occasion my wishes were, I felt, more relevant than hers. Would I feel disloyal? Would it feel wrong? I decided to give it a trial and see, and on that basis Muriel and I started our bridge partnership.

Keeping up hobbies and interests is important. It's important for children and for friends to realise that they have a part to play in encouraging you to try to keep up your hobbies and interests. It's equally important for you to respond to the encouragement, and not reject it.

Most stroke victims recover, but some, like Dilys, do not. In either case, the surviving relative will need the support of a familiar hobby more than ever. Activities which involve interaction with other people (like bridge) may be more important than solitary activities (like gardening) since it is too easy for relatives to withdraw from society when they have to take care of a discharged patient or recover from a bereavement. Everyone needs to lick their wounds. But at some time everyone has to emerge from the den, and it's easier to do so if we've made regular forays than if we've sat inside waiting until the wounds have healed permanently.

Both sons returned from their week's holiday, saying they'd come up to see their mother.

"Don't take time off work specially," I said. "Come up at the weekend. If there's any change in Mum's condition before then, I'll let you know at once."

Both came at the weekend, and went back as usual on the Sunday.

By the middle of the last week in September the nurses said that Dilys was a lot weaker. Patients on water apparently only lived for about six weeks. She had now already exceeded that limit.

"It'll be days, not weeks," the nurse said.

Sister came into Dilys's room for one of her regular visits and tenderly smoothed Dilys forehead and hair. I'd seen her comforting and cheering patients so many times over the last few months. How did she manage to give so much sympathy to so many of her charges, I wondered. In the corridor outside, she confirmed the nurse's view.

"I'm afraid poor Dilys is just skin and bone now. I'm astonished she's still with us."

"She's always had a strong heart, and of course she's had wonderful nursing," I replied. To my surprise Sister seemed quite touched.

My own feelings were mixed. I was pleased that Dilys showed no reactions at all: no pain, no suffering. Yet I'd soon not be seeing her again. In spite of her lifeless condition, that was a hard situation to accept. How would I react, I wondered. How could I imagine the depth of sorrow? Would I feel relief? And would I feel guilt at that?

The last weeks

The weather was changing. When it was too cool, or too damp to sit in the little nature reserve and eat lunch, I ate it in the car, or bought lunch in a small café. The warm summer days were now a memory, the leaves were beginning to turn, and there was an occasional autumn nip in the morning air. The summer was dying.

One morning at the end of September Dilys was beginning to struggle. Her breathing was hampered by the phlegm that accumulated in her throat, and which she was unable to swallow. The nurses paid regular visits, using suction to dispel the fluid. I felt anxious: yet by the afternoon she was more relaxed, sleeping quietly again.

Sister caught me as I was leaving.

"Michael rang me to say he intended visiting this evening, driving over after work."

This was unexpected.

"He may have meant it as a surprise," she said.

Nevertheless I rang Michael's wife, who explained that as he'd been abroad over the weekend and hadn't seen his Mum, he wanted to come over today. I felt pleased.

He arrived at the house at nine o'clock, straight from the hospital, with news that Dilys wasn't so well. The water had been reduced, too, and he'd arranged to ring the hospital at 10 o'clock that evening.

The night staff were calm and definite: there'd been no change over the last few hours.

"Should we come and stay overnight?" I asked.

"I don't really feel that's necessary," the nurse said. "But I don't want you to keep away from the hospital if you feel you want to come. The guest room is yours, any time."

I thought for a moment

"We'll ring you at once if there's any change," she promised, but added that it was always possible that Dilys's breathing might just stop in the night.

We decided to take the nurse's advice.

When Michael left for work at six o'clock, the situation was unchanged. I continued with my regular visits for the next two days. Dilys was obviously very weak. I noticed that the curtains across the glass door into her room were now firmly drawn.

Then on the morning of the third day, the hospital rang before I left for my visit.

"There's been a change overnight," the nurse said. "You may want to let your family know, in case they want to come."

I rang the two sons and Janet in New Zealand. Michael arrived later that morning and John came up from Birmingham in the afternoon. Janet was holding an open ticket.

All that long day we sat by the bedside, taking turns to walk outside and to eat.

"Just let us know when you'd like a cup of tea or coffee," the nurses insisted, and a tray appeared and reappeared regularly.

It was nearly midnight when her breathing became very irregular. Suddenly her blind eyes opened as if she wanted to see her family for the last time; then they closed and she seemed to subside gently into the pillow, as if the effort had been too much. For nearly half an hour she breathed more quietly and peacefully than for days. And then the breathing stopped, just stopped.

October

Dilys had wanted a humanitarian funeral. We'd both sat through too many occasions when well-meaning clerics delivered hollow eulogies on people they hardly knew, attempting unsuccessfully to capture their remembered talents in thin pencil sketches. On this last appearance a loved relative deserves to be displayed as a rich portrait in oils, painted by someone close and familiar. So between some of Dilys's favourite music, John and I both gave short addresses: a diptych, to continue the metaphor.

For me she would always be the strong, loving centre of the family, her firm views providing the guidance the children needed; yet she was such a mischievous person, with the quickest, most amusing repartee. I would always think of her on a sunny afternoon, pottering happily in her garden, floppy sun hat on, stopping to chat to all who passed by.

The many friends filed by. The wake was a cheerful event, just as she would have wished, relations and friends making the most of the opportunity to renew acquaintances. And then the last mourner went and the day ended. I suddenly felt very tired.

I missed the regular visits to Dilys. So far the days had filled themselves with essential activities. Now that the funeral was over, her clothes sent to charities, the children dispersed to their families and their work, the marvellous little hospital thanked, I determined to continue to fill my time in every possible way. I'd forgotten about Bob, but I suddenly felt I wanted to see how he was getting on.

Bob was fine, and pleased to see me. He was slowly recovering greater control of his damaged functions and his speech, though not perfect, was much more intelligible. He still had some difficulties with actions that to most of us are so everyday that they are automatic – picking up dropped articles, putting toothpaste on a brush, for example. But overall, improvement was good.

Many devices are available for helping with the problems of everyday living for those who are recovering from strokes. For the two simple examples given above there are implements for picking things up from the floor without bending and toothbrush holders for easy charging with toothpaste. The Disabled Living Foundation offers over 50 leaflets giving information about the various aids to independent living and the choices available. These include information about helpful clothing, continence aids, putting on footwear, useful telephones, wheelchair choices etc. etc. – all that someone recovering from the effects of a stroke might need.

I noticed the grab rails at strategic points in the hallway and bathroom.

"The occupational therapist arranged for these," he said. "Most useful," he added.

Back at the house, there were many invitations for me to stay with relatives and friends, but for the moment I wanted to stay in the familiar surroundings of the home we'd shared. For days I was occupied with the paper work and the formalities that followed. At the time they were a chore, but looking back, there is advantage in having procedures and tasks to keep the bereaved busy.

Not everyone wants to deal themselves with the many procedures that follow a bereavement, and many prefer to hand matters over to a solicitor. What is important is to be busy; some may want to arrange a holiday; others may want to take up long deferred projects; others may prefer to work through the unavoidable rituals themselves.

I handled the arrangements for gaining probate for the will and for the execution of Dilys's wishes. This was an interesting legal education, gained through many phone calls and letters. It was a lengthy process, lasting many weeks, but not as difficult as I had feared. So many offices had clearly put particularly sympathetic staff on duty to provide helpful answers to enquiries from bereaved people.

One phone call had a particular impact. Yet another return call from one of my enquiries, I thought. But it wasn't dry business; the central tissue donation agency was on the phone. Tissue donation! I'd forgotten all about that. The lady in charge thanked me gently for agreeing to donate tissue, chatted for a moment or two to put me at my ease, and then asked would I mind answering a few questions about any illnesses Dilys had had during her lifetime. She apologised for the enquiry, explaining the reasons in a very understanding way. I thought of the occasional medical events that had punctuated our 53 years together, and relayed them to the caller.

The pictures of happier days which stood around the rooms at home were constantly reminding me of the great life we'd had together, beginning to place a protective cover over the wounds of the last few months. Memories, not just of the ups and downs of Dilys's life, but also of the last days in hospital were beginning to weaken. But that enquiry brought them back.

My mind returned to that day in May, six months ago, just before the stroke, when Dilys and I were walking through the town, intending to buy a pair of sandals. With a wrench in my gut I realised that we hadn't bought them, and now we never would.

A week later the tissue centre rang again.

"I thought you ought to know that we've considered what you told us, and since we have to be very careful over transplanted tissue, we decided that it would be wiser not to use any material from Dilys."

Be prepared for that possible outcome too. An offer to donate tissue, doesn't mean that the offer will be taken up. Since the offer to donate tissue is usually made long before the moment arrives, this outcome cannot be predicted. Who can forecast the condition of our bodies in years to come? But of course it's always possible that your decision will make a wonderful difference to someone else's life.

I felt vaguely disappointed: all that emotional struggle to no effect – Dilys would have been disappointed too. But it was another chapter closed. I put the phone down.

First week of November

The doorbell rang. Surprise: the doctor! Was there some mistake?

"Just called to see how you're getting on."

He came in and sat down in the study, where I was wrestling with the paperwork involved in obtaining probate on Dilys's will. I got coffee for the two of us.

"Managing all right? We always call to check on bereaved patients, just to see how they're doing."

I felt a surge of gratitude. The news was full of the Iraq war, people being blown to bits and maimed for life, and yet here was more evidence of the basic goodness in humanity. Back to his question.

"Yes, I'm coping well." I gestured at the desk. "I'm busy with paper work. But I'm starting my hobbies, again. And friends and family have been wonderful."

He nodded. "It's a month, now, since your wife died."

A month: fancy the practice noticing that. "Yes. I've read it takes a couple of years to get over things like this."

He looked thoughtful. "You'll never really get over it, you know. But you'll adjust to it, accommodate to it."

"I'm trying to. I've asked a friend to stay, and he's coming tomorrow."

I first met Jack at a climbing weekend over half a century ago, and we'd seen each other from time to time over the years. Our climbing days were long over, and latterly, our activities together consisted almost entirely of meeting at the annual mountaineering club dinner. His wife, Mary, had died about a fortnight before Dilys, and as the date for this year's dinner was approaching, and the venue was close by, I'd asked him to stay with me. Breakfast and lunch would be easy, and we could go to the dinner together, two widowers, company for each other.

Friends and neighbours call in to see how you're getting on – as the doctor did. But if you've lost your partner, there is an unavoidable emptiness in the house: the silence can become oppressive. The voices of radio and television help, but someone staying in the house, a human presence, offering company, if only for a day or two, can lift the spirits.

After Dilys died, it was strange to realise how much I missed doing things for her: I hadn't expected that reaction. Having a visitor to stay makes you think again about someone else's needs, and that helps to bring back a more normal feeling.

It's better to start slowly. So think of someone you know who won't be a pain, and ask just for a night or two, not for weeks. It's worth considering eating the main meals out, or using ready meals. Jack brought a sleeping bag, so there was no problem with providing linen. Make the first visit easy!

"Good." The doctor approved. We talked for another 10 minutes or so, and he left, telling me to be sure to make an appointment if I felt concerned about anything.

Jack arrived, his car boot full of enough food and alcohol for a week. The club dinner went well, and the next morning I put in a load of washing. Washing was the easiest of chores; just load the machine, same setting every time, and when it finished whack the clothes in the tumble dryer for 90 minutes at full heat. No problem.

I'd never understood why Dilys spent so much time ironing. Why iron things like underwear, pyjamas, sheets, when the moment you used them, they rumpled? Shirts were drip-dry these days, and even they needn't be ironed. My slogan for housewives had always been "Abolish ironing!" And now that I was o.c. washing clothes, that's exactly what I did.

As I loaded the machine that morning, Jack was watching carefully. I poured the powder and liquid into their respective compartments, and switched on.

"So that's what you do," he commented.

"Don't you?" I asked, surprised.

"No: I've got to learn what to do. Mary always took care of the washing."

It was six weeks since Mary had died. "You haven't been doing the washing by hand, Jack, have you?"

He looked shamefaced. "No, I haven't been washing at all, just working my way through my wardrobe."

The partners of stroke victims are often elderly, and for them, readjusting to life without a partner can be especially hard, particularly for a widower. The elderly have spent their married lives in a different society, one that believed that it made sense to divide the tasks of daily living, men handling the more technical and heavy jobs around the house and garden, while the women managed the essential household chores, including the washing and cooking.

How times have changed! Many new widowers, like me, have to learn or relearn basic survival skills after over half a century of being looked after. But there aren't any courses to help them: there should be, I thought.

One newly widowed friend wanted guidance over using the microwave. By now, I'd met several widowers who'd been managing on their own for quite some time. Why not get together to exchange tips? Widows have no problems with living skills, though they might need help with replacing tap washers and handling the finances. But widowers need help, not just on microwaves, but on generally managing on their own.

So we meet once a month for a beer and sandwich lunch at a local pub. Yes, we do funny things we never thought we'd do, like exchanging recipes, and learning about cleaning equipment, but we mainly talk about the football results and local politics. More importantly, we enjoy a social occasion.

Not far away lived a lady whom we knew as 'the dog walker'. Every day she passed the house at least once, and often several times, always with a dog at the end of a leash. The dogs weren't the same, and we'd learnt that she enjoyed dog walking, and walked other people's dogs beside her own. The dog walker always said a very pleasant 'hello' when I met her, but this afternoon she stopped, and asked how I was managing.

"I haven't said anything before," she added sympathetically, "since I know some people can get upset if anyone intrudes on their private grief."

"I'm managing well, thanks. And it's kind of you to ask." We chatted for a minute or two, until her eager hound saw a labrador up the road and dragged her away for a social visit to his old friend. I realised I'd not had the prickle behind the eyes, nor the lump in the throat. I'd managed to talk about my situation rationally, and not emotionally. Was this progress? Was I accommodating to it? I felt encouraged.

I called on Bob again. In the pressure of the last few months I'd almost forgotten about Bob and his stroke. Tucked away in a corner were a couple of computers. A large Spanish dictionary lay open on a chair.

I took him out to get some shopping and for coffee. His walking was limited, but he could manage a hundred yards or so with the help of an arm. His speech was definitely better. Carers provided via social services visited regularly, a lady came weekly to help clean, and he had meals on wheels. He was still being seen by the hospital stroke team, but the appointments were much less frequent now.

"I'm not going to improve much more." Did he sound a little sorry for himself, I wondered.

"But they all say I've done well, and I'm pleased with the improvement. The move to the flats has been a great help." No, he sounded positive.

Perhaps the best feature of his life was the range of activities he enjoyed. The scrabble club in the flats, the book club he'd joined, the occasional slide shows and entertainments, the visitors who called, all helped to fill in his time. I asked about the computers.

"One's my old one, and the new one my sons bought me when I came out of hospital."

"Do you use it much?" I asked.

"Years ago I wrote a small handbook of useful phrases and idioms in Spanish. I'm surprised that it continues to sell" – he gave a grin at the thought – " and even more surprised that the publishers have asked for a new edition, together with proverbs this time. I've promised it for next summer, in time for the holiday rush."

I congratulated him. Getting published at 85 was pretty marvellous. The dictionary now made sense.

"I enjoy working at it," Bob said. "I only do a little at a time, but it gives me a purpose."

How right Bob was. It really is important for stroke victims to find a task, an interest that involves them once recovery is on the way. It needn't, like Bob's, be an intellectual activity; many people find a practical interest that suits them. The occupational therapist can help with ideas, but encouragement and support from relatives are often the keys to getting the convalescent started. Discharge from hospital does not mean that the relatives can relax. Now is the time when they are more needed than ever.

It was his positive attitude that impressed me more than the physical improvement. The early depression had all gone, and he had a purpose, an objective, something he could achieve.

Poor Dilys had a very different stroke, and I had a very different situation to deal with. Accommodate to it: I thought back to the doctor's visit. It was now over a month since Dilys had died, and in a reassuring flood of confidence I remembered the hospitality I'd received over the summer. I'd been shown so much warmth, received so many dinner invitations. I decided I wanted to start to repay the kindnesses. I'll join the world again; I'll start entertaining! Not just a meal out, but a proper dinner. Who to ask back?

The couple, old friends, who'd given me a meal so many times; they were the obvious first choice. Don't hesitate, I said to myself: your resolution might weaken. I rang them at once, and fixed a date. Committed. Now I'll have to go through with it; no pulling out. There ought to be a fourth; and the fourth ought to be a single lady, to balance the group. Now there's a delicate problem. Among Dilys's circle of women friends were several widows and spinsters. All had been solicitous and caring over the summer, but none of them had offered to show me how to use the washing machine, or offered to cook a meal for me. Of course not; any offer might have been misunderstood, misinterpreted; I appreciated that. Still, there shouldn't be any misunderstanding over asking Vera, an old friend of Dilys's to make up a small dinner party. She talked well and we all knew each other in various contexts. I rang her. A slight but definite pause.

"It's to make up a four for dinner, with…" and I named the couple coming.

"How brave of you," Vera exclaimed, "can I help you?" I felt more apprehensive than brave, but I was going to manage this myself.

"No thanks," I said.

I now had a challenge – I had to prepare dinner for four, something I'd never done before. It would be an important milestone in my new life. In a strange way I felt Dilys would be watching to see how I coped. So I would cope, for her sake as well as mine.

I spent the next few days deciding what to cook. First thought: it would have to be easy; something I could prepare beforehand and just put in the oven before the guests came. I couldn't offer my usual fare; a ready meal, or a pizza. No, to show my appreciation for all the support I'd had from my friends, I'd cook something a bit more special. I tried to recall what Dilys used to prepare. A casserole, I thought; she made great casseroles. That should fill the bill. Where were the recipes?

I found Dilys's recipe book. I opened it for the first time, ever. The first pages held a few lovingly written descriptions of dishes she used to prepare at the start of our lives together, recipes from half a century ago. There was arctic wonder, holyrood cake – great family parties came to mind: birthdays, Christmases, events long gone. I felt an additional sadness at seeing the familiar writing again, and I turned the pages, looking for casseroles. Nothing suitable here. Most of the recipes were scribbled on bits of paper and card, tucked into the leaves of the book in a system that must have meant something to Dilys, but flummoxed me. No sign of a casserole recipe.

I turned to one of her cookery books, and looked up casseroles. Beef? No, might worry people. Lamb? Seemed a messy recipe. Pork? That looked easier. Pork casserole it would be. Better try it out first. I bought the ingredients the next day, found an apron, and put it on. What a charley I looked! More importantly, I summarised the procedure on a card, and started my own little library of recipes. I felt I'd made a beginning, opened up a new front in the struggle, so to speak. Masquerading as a chef, at my time of life!

Judging by the delicious taste, the trial run went well, I thought. But what to do with the rest of the casserole? It wouldn't be enough for the dinner party; could I use it again myself? Wasn't there some funny business about reheating meat dishes? So many things to learn about this cooking business. I suddenly thought of the TV show, 'Who Wants to be a Millionaire?' If you can't answer a question, phone a friend. So I phoned a friend.

"Divide it into single portions and freeze them," she advised. And then you can reheat each one when you want it. Excellent! That way I'd have three ready home cooked meals in store, so to speak. Ha! Another lesson learnt.

The sweet: an attempt a few weeks before to make a pie with pastry had ended in disaster. "Crumbles are really easy," a friend had said. I'd not believed her the first time, when I'd used a fork to mix the topping, and the mess was horrible. I'd since learnt to use the forks that nature gave us: our fingers.

There were frozen raspberries in the freezer from Dilys's last active summer, nearly two years ago, and I could stew apples. So we'd have a raspberry and apple crumble, with ice cream of course. Sounded good. But the big problem would be the timing. I had to ensure that the vegetables and the casserole and the crumble were all ready at the right time. Back to memories of work schedules and planning. I made a flowsheet. It looked like the timetable for a military operation.

5.00 Lay table
5.20 Oven on
5.30 Casserole in
5.45 Sherry glasses and nibbles out
5.55 Potatoes to boil
6.00 Guests arrive

and so on....

Get hold of 'Recipes for Disasters' (see the list) before you start, a book which advises on how to deal with cooking emergencies, and take heart from realising how many other would be chefs have had to make unexpected adaptations.

Don't worry about possible failures – a possible problem with the meal really makes a friendly dinner party go with a swing. Guests love trying to help an inexperienced host, so have a go.

Surprise! It worked. We had a great evening, and my guests stayed till 11 o'clock. The food may not have been cordon bleu, but at least they all could say nice things about it. I looked at the kitchen, something like London after an air raid, with bits of dishes, half empty wineglasses, crumpled napkins and other rubbish strewn all round. Leave the clearing up till the morning, I thought, suddenly feeling tired. Tired but strangely pleased. I went to sleep remembering what my visitors had said as they went.

"Dilys would have been proud of you."

Survivorland

The first Christmas began to approach, and I began to realise how different it would be. For so many years we'd decorated the tree together, now I had to do this myself. We'd put up the cards together, read the messages from friends together, bought the presents together. Now I had to deal with the cards and presents myself. The picture of my life was changing after the summer of the stroke.

Being a single, and not one of a couple, was different in so many ways. My patterns of friendship began slowly to change. You live in survivorland, now, I told myself. It's inhabited by a vast number of singles – mainly widows, widowers, divorcees, the separated – all living on their own. Your address is still the same, but the country is different: its habits are not the same, it lives by slightly different social codes. It's not easy to ask a couple in to join you for an evening, as you used to; three is an odd number.

Suvivorland is also mainly female. This was strikingly brought home to me at the bridge club dinner I attended. There were three married couples in the group of 24, and of the remaining 18, I was the only male: the rest were single females.

I was relieved when Michael and family asked me to stay with them over that first Christmas. They couldn't have been kinder, and being in a jolly family certainly eased the strangeness of my first Christmas as a single, after over 50 years as one of a couple. Even so, there were occasional poignant moments. I particularly remember the six year old grandson – a joy, enthusiastic and lively. He'd had a lot of presents, including a racing car. One day he stopped it, looked up at me and suddenly said, sadly,

"Why did Nain have to die?"

Why, indeed? He'd been so fond of his Grandmother, and they'd been such great friends. How to reply? This was the first close relationship he'd lost, and he wanted the pain explained in terms a six year old would understand. It was important to get it right, not to try to conceal the reality of death, yet not to worry him with possible fears that a child's mind might construct.

"She died because she was very ill," I said, and went on to explain that although everybody has to die sometime, no one else he knew was likely to die just then, not for a very very long time.

I waited for more questions, expecting him to ask where she'd gone, but "Your turn with the red car, Granpa," he said, cheerful again. The explanation had satisfied him for the moment, and later, I told his parents about our little conversation. They needed to know what he was thinking about and to be prepared for more questions.

It's not only adults who feel shocked when a family member has a stroke; children are upset too. Since so many strokes happen to older people, grandchildren are frequently involved, and grandchildren often do have a very warm and special relationship with their grandparents. A stroke may well be something children have never met before, and they want to understand what has happened, why their relative's speech is suddenly poor, why movement has been affected, and so on. It's important to remember their needs, and to try to explain the situation in words that match their age and understanding.

Some children may feel so shocked that they clam up and say nothing, feeling overwhelmed by this sudden, unimaginable change in a person they are fond of. It's then more important than ever to talk gently to them about the stroke, and to help and encourage them to tell you about the worries they have. There are publications (for example, 'Grandpa's had a Stroke' – published by the Stroke Association, details in the list) that give guidance, aiming to help children who need to know what this strange and worrying event – a stroke – means.

Bereavement after a stroke raises other problems. Older children have some understanding of the concept of death, whereas young children, without experience of death, need help to understand what's happened.

All these points face older relatives when they themselves are under pressure and are trying to cope with changes to their own lives. It's not an easy time. Nevertheless it really is important to remember the children; they need support too.

Shortly after Christmas I had a special message from our daughter (or should I say 'my daughter' now: that's another delicate issue. If you use 'our', then people who don't know you usually assume that you have a wife and may ask about her. For a short while, that hurts.) At the end of January, son-in-law was going to be away at work, and Janet, who was working part time herself, would be on her own in New Zealand with the children. They would be on holiday: would I come and help? Would I? Another holiday to look forward to! On second thoughts, perhaps more of a responsibility than a holiday... But I booked my ticket at once.

When we'd been out to see Janet previously, we'd always been away for five or six weeks. No point in going all that way for less. But on my own? I felt that I needed to see how I'd manage in a different household, even though it was my daughter's. So I booked for a fortnight, just enough to cover her over the time when she'd be coping with the children on her own. A sort of long distance childsitting.

In the plane on the return journey, I thought over the holiday. It had been a long time since I'd been responsible for adolescents, and this had been a reminder of the skills involved in coping with them. They'd been pretty tolerant of their grandfather, I thought, and we'd had a couple of chats about Dilys. It had been a good break in the sun, but a fortnight was long enough; I needed to return to familiar territory. Next time, I'd stay longer.

Time for more entertaining. I added up the various friends who'd fed me over the past year; far too many to have round for meals. It would have to be a party, the first I'd done on my own. We'd held many parties in our lives together, and I smiled as I thought of the curry party for 28 friends that Dilys had once done.

"I'm cheating," she said, buying 15 curried chicken meals from a well known supermarket, and putting the lot in a large saucepan. "I hope they won't guess."

They didn't, and cheating or not, it had been a great success.

But I couldn't do anything like that myself. It would have to be a lunchtime party, I decided; people wouldn't stay as long as at a dinner, and I needn't provide so much food. So in the spring, nearly a year after Dilys had been taken ill, I invited twenty friends round to drinks and light refreshments, buying the refreshments from caterers. Once I'd got over the work of rearranging the furniture in the rooms, the actual party worked well; guests went round with the plates while I filled and refilled their glasses. I went to bed that night feeling pleased; I'd repaid some of the hospitality I owed, and the house had been a cheerful place again. Another hurdle overcome.

It was nearly six months since Dilys had died. I still felt numbed, and after the stress of that long summer, and the paper work that had followed across the winter, I felt I needed a holiday, a real holiday, not staying with the family. I certainly wasn't going to holiday on my own – that would be the last experience I wanted: I needed company. So I booked a long weekend's walking holiday in the Lake District with a group. Another widower friend was interested, and in the end the two of us went. The weather was good, the walking enjoyable, and the group was friendly.

It wasn't quite the first holiday I'd had without Dilys. During our married life there had been a few occasions when it had made more sense for either she or I to spend a break without the other, but then the other one had always been there to return to. And it was returning home that brought the sudden pain: walking up to the closed door, opening it to the silent rooms, and realising that I was returning to an empty house, not a home. The difference was something I'd have to get used to. But there was no doubt – I felt much better for the weekend.

Holidays are important. It's wise to plan ahead, perhaps not as meticulously as another widower friend, who'd arranged three or four holidays a year for the next few years. Any break from routine, even just one day away, is something to plan for, something to look forward to, a shaft of sunshine to lighten the shadows. It's better to think of a holiday with others, if at all possible, either with a friend or in a group. Groups of like minded holidaymakers are usually friendly and there are likely to be others in similar situations to yours.

Think of anniversaries, too. Do you want to be at home for an important anniversary, or would it be better to be away? Work around that when you make your bookings.

Michael rang in May.

"Where in the world would you like to go, Dad? What would you like to see?"

What a question! My thoughts raced from the Canaries to the Nile, Iceland, the Karakoram... "Yosemite," I said. This wonderful valley in western USA, the original National Park, the home of unmatched scenery and of extreme rock-climbing, that was where I'd like to go.

"Why?" I added.

"Because we'll go there then," Michael enthused. "I'm finishing my job and starting another a fortnight later. So at the end of this month I've got free time, a dispensation from my wife, and so I'm taking you to Yosemite for a 10 day walking holiday." I could almost see the broad grin on his face. I was taken aback. I hadn't had a holiday with the children since our family holidays over a quarter of a century ago.

What an experience! Michael made all the arrangements, and for the first time for over half a century I didn't have to book anything. I recalled the times when the children were young and Dilys and I had taken them on holiday – camping on the continent, farmhouses in west Wales, rented accommodation in Scotland. Now the roles were reversed: I was being taken on holiday, and it was highly enjoyable. Not only was the scenery magnificent, but just having 10 days with a son as sole companion was a revelation in itself. I realised how close we still were after those years in which he'd left home, married, and raised his own family.

The first anniversary of Dilys's death approached. She hadn't said where she wanted her ashes scattered, and a year ago, I had decided on the place. Before we married we'd spent several holidays in North Wales, staying in a small cottage in one of the valleys. The cottage was reached from the road by a footpath that crossed the little river and then ran past a large rock. The rock featured in many school geography textbooks as a fine example of glaciation, and as it was the halfway point on the path, we'd often rested our heavy packs there and admired the view. The rock, the valley and the mountains held many happy memories, and it was there that Michael and I had emptied the urn to the winds. I knew she would have been pleased.

I went back there on the anniversary. Once again I sat on the rock, thought of Dilys and the half century that had passed, listened to the river and the wind, and watched the cloud shadows march across the mountains. For a moment, I thought I heard her voice again, and then I lost it on the moving air. I felt the sadness. Yet as I sat there, I also felt strangely at ease, not wanting to leave, attached.

It started to rain, and the spell broke. I walked back; not happy, but very glad I'd been there.

When my widower friend and I had holidayed in the Lake District, in the spring, we'd met up with a couple of congenial widows from the south coast. Although we hadn't seen anything of each other in the day, we'd often sat together for meals, and enjoyed each other's company in the evenings. When the holiday ended, we said we ought to meet again. Holiday friendships often end at the end of the holiday, in spite of vows to meet again, but on this occasion the friendships didn't end, and the four of us met again for an autumn walking weekend in the Cotswolds.

Isabella was a few years younger than me, and had been widowed for more than 10 years. I found her a very attractive companion, easy to talk to, quiet, independent, and with a gentle sense of humour. I spent that second Christmas with John and family, and this time I felt strong enough to spend a whole week away. Isabella lived close enough for me to visit for one of the days, and we enjoyed a very happy walk together. Instead of resting on the stern of the ship, watching the distant shoreline fading, I feel I am now standing on the prow, heading through new seas, to new horizons.

We arranged to join a group for a spring holiday.

I took stock of my life. In May, it would be two years since Dilys had her stroke, two years in which I'd managed on my own. In some ways my life was very full. I could certainly cope with the basic skills of running the house. I had many different activities: two bridge clubs, a writing circle, a men's lunch club, bowls, badminton and table tennis groups, occasional driving for meals on wheels, taking walks for the Ramblers and for the Walking for Health group, Bob to visit, the local National Trust Association, a leisure centre committee.... Too many activities I sometimes thought. Yes, I could indeed live in survivorland, but there was an emptiness, a gap which Dilys had once occupied. Her place could never be filled, but I remembered her attitude when, as all married couples do, we'd discussed how the other would manage when one of us died.

"You find someone else," she said. "Full permission granted – I'd be happier knowing you were not on your own."

That possibility had only fleetingly crossed my mind up to now. I was on friendly terms with a number of ladies, a lively bridge partner; a friendly near neighbour whom we'd known for nearly 20 years; a compatible member of our writing circle with a similar outlook on life; and Isabella. I was on friendly terms with all four, but no relationship had progressed beyond friendship. Isabella and I have similar interests (and some different ones), and similar experiences – we have both lost our partners. It suddenly struck me that we also seemed to get on extremely well.

So now the summer has come round again, the second summer after the summer of the stroke. Isabella and I are going on a holiday on our own in order to see how our relationship progresses. It is now over two years since Dilys had her stroke, and it will soon be two years since she died. I've come through the greatest trauma of my life, losing my partner. Yet, like everyone who has travelled along the same roller coaster, the journey does end, and the stressful memories begin to fade. There is a new, a different life to be lived, whether on your own or not, a life that has to be seized. Yes, the memories of the old life do begin to fade, but they never disappear. And once in a while, when I'm on my own in the house, I'll switch on the CD player, and listen again to 'The Ashokan Farewell.'

Useful contacts

We've put together a short list of useful organisations to contact if you or someone you know has had a stroke. As contact details often change we've put the list on our website where it can be regularly updated, rather than print it here. You can find the list at **www.whiteladderpress.com**; click on 'useful contacts' next to the information about this book.

If you don't have access to the Internet you can contact White Ladder Press by any of the means listed on the following page and we'll print off a hard copy and post it to you free of charge.

Contact us

You're welcome to contact White Ladder Press if you have any questions or comments for either us or the author. Please use whichever of the following routes suits you.

Phone: 01803 813343 between 9am and 5.30pm

Email: enquiries@whiteladderpress.com

Fax: 01803 813928

Address: White Ladder Press, Great Ambrook, Near Ipplepen, Devon TQ12 5UL

Website: **www.whiteladderpress.com**

What can our website do for you?

If you want more information about any of our books, you'll find it at **www.whiteladderpress.com**. In particular you'll find extracts from each of our books, and reviews of those that are already published. We also run special offers on future titles if you order online before publication. And you can request a copy of our free catalogue.

Many of our books also have links pages, useful addresses and so on relevant to the subject of the book. You'll also find out a bit more about us and, if you're a writer yourself, you'll find our submission guidelines for authors. So please check us out and let us know if you have any comments, questions or suggestions.

Want any more useful books?

If you've found this book useful, how about reading another of our books which will help stroke sufferers? On the next few pages you'll find extracts from two of our other books: **Surviving a Stroke** *Recovering and adjusting to living with hypertension* and **Stop Smoking, Stay Cool** *A dedicated smoker's guide to not smoking.*

The first extract is from *Surviving a Stroke* by Mike Ripley. At the age of 50, Mike had a stroke. This is his story of the stroke itself and the next year in the recovery process, together with a mass of practical tips and advice for anyone else recovering from stroke. As a comic crime thriller writer, Mike Ripley looks for the humour in any situation, and finds it even in this one.

If you'd like to order a copy of the book, it costs £7.99 and is available via any of the routes on page 166, or you can use the order form at the back of this book.

Surviving a Stroke

Recovering and adjusting to living with hypertension

MIKE RIPLEY

Extract from Chapter 5

The Great Escape

The first part of my escape plan is to reclaim as much normalcy as possible; to do things I would normally do and not just sit around waiting for something to happen or a bolt out of the blue to make me fit again. I must not lie there and accept it. I must not play by the rules the stroke wants to impose on me.

In my first days in The Twilight Zone, Alyson had smuggled in my mobile phone, but as there are signs everywhere in the hospital warning that phone signals could interfere with medical equipment, I have not even switched it on. But from D-Bay's window I can see people in the snow-covered car park below using them, so I decide to join them.

Hiding the phone in the pocket of my dressing gown, I walk through Birch Ward and out on to the stairwell without being stopped, searched or questioned by anyone (though there is no reason why anyone should – patients are free to move about and visitors come and go all day).

I experience a great feeling of accomplishment, having got out of D-Bay and then out of Birch Ward entirely, but as I am on the top floor, there is nowhere else to go but down and so I do, confidently taking the stairs rather than the lift. Holding tightly on to the hand rail fixed in the wall, I lower myself like a mountaineer down two short flights until I find I am on the First Floor where the stairwell has one of the biggest vending machines I have ever seen, fully stocked with crisps and chocolate bars of all known flavours and brands. I immediately kick myself for not bringing any cash with me, as Alyson has left me a pile of change for newspapers and the phone-box on the ward (which still isn't working, as it is full and won't take any more coins).

It never occurs to me, at least not then, that everything in that machine is loaded either with salt or sugar (probably both) – the very things we overweight hypertensives will be warned against.

Down two more flights and I'm on the ground floor and there are automatic doors leading to the outside world and I've made it. I am standing in the hospital car park. I'm in pyjamas, dressing gown and slippers and it is snowing. I suddenly realise I feel very cold, very foolish and I have my mobile phone clutched in my right hand but I cannot remember for the life of me who it was I wanted to call.

There is no one else in sight. In fact, the snow is coming down so thickly I can't see the main hospital about fifty yards away. Then a car looking for a parking slot goes into a skid and

Texas, and teaches people to be speech therapists. Both person-ally and professionally he has experience of heart problems and strokes, and has been emailing for a diagnosis since it happened.

I tell Aly to reply with the words "right side – clot, not bleed" only, which she does and he responds with: "You have, my friend, avoided a very bad bullet".

Stop Smoking, Stay Cool

A dedicated smoker's guide to not smoking

RICHARD CRAZE

Any stroke sufferer who smokes will be strongly advised to give up. It's easy to say, but much harder to do. *Stop Smoking, Stay Cool* is Richard Craze's honest and funny account of giving up smoking after dedicating himself to tobacco for over 30 years. His journal holds the reader's hand through withdrawal symptoms, mood swings, coughs, mouth ulcers and all the other symptoms, including The Voice. He offers real help for those wanting to give up, and especially those who see smoking as cool (which is, frankly, most smokers) and don't want to sacrifice their personal image when they quit the fags.

If you'd like to order a copy of the book, it costs £7.99 and is available via any of the routes on page 166, or you can use the order form at the back of this book.

Stop Smoking, Stay Cool

DAY 20

As I approach the end of my first three weeks without tobacco I am questioning my identity as a 'not smoking at the moment thank you' sort of person. I mean, who is this new smelling of soap chap I have become? When I smoked I was a smoker; that was me. I smoked roll ups. I smelt of tobacco and tweed and damp corduroy. I was relaxed and chilled. I wore John Lennon glasses and read Stephen King and liked a nice cup of tea (mind you I am drinking upwards of twenty cups a day now; is that another addiction I shall have to address in time?) and walking my dogs across fields where I could lean on a farm gate and have a roll up and watch the clouds and internally philosophise about life and death and the universe and everything.

Now I am sharp with the children, cold and fresh, smelling of carbolic, afraid to sit still for too long in case I give in to this damn ridiculous voice in my head, unable to work or sleep, eating too much, a neurotic bundle of twitches and jerks. I mean, who am I now? Do I approve of who I have become? Am I the sort of person I wouldn't have shared a railway carriage with before? Have I become a New Man? I liked the old me, the smelly, slightly singed around the edges me. I have become...no, I can't say it...I have become...a non smoker. Arg! I can hear the Voice mocking me.

You see smoking is so attractive. Smoking is rebellious, young, carefree. It makes such a defiant statement about who you are. If you smoke you are signing up to wearing a leather jacket with the collar turned up, listening to rock and roll, staying up late, talking about life, the universe and everything, rebelling and behaving like a grown up. Now you are washed and ready for bed after your tea. You are a child again. You smell nice, but of nothing real or grown up or dangerous. You have gone from being James Dean to Wendy Craig in one swift stubbing out of a fag. You are a disappointment to me.

And to myself. I could almost weaken. This is such a persuasive argument. I could, almost. I do like the idea of smoking a pipe. I've always thought the smell of damp tweed and pipe tobacco a good thing.

My grandfather smoked roll ups. He had a silver tobacco tin with a sun burst engraved on it. How do I remember it so clearly? I have it by me as I write. My uncle gave it to me to remember Pop by. I used it for many years myself but it is now redundant. Pop died of emphysema/bronchitis/pneumonia, due to his smoking, at the age of sixty eight. I don't think a day goes by when I don't think of him and miss him. I didn't have a father so my grandfather was the nearest I got to a role model/father figure. Is this why I have smoked so long, so often, so much? I have to question it. To beat this Voice I have to know why I smoked.

My grandfather rolled roll ups gently, with time and care and, as a small boy, I would watch him fascinated, hypnotised, in rapture. I loved the smell of them, of him. It's easy now to remember the hawking cough which I blanked at the time, and the fact that it was smoking which killed him. It also killed my mother at the age of seventy. Did she smoke because her beloved dad did? Were we all trying to be like Pop? To be Pop? He was the kindest, funniest man ever. We all loved him.

Notice how the Voice goes quiet when the serious business of smoking comes up? When we talk of death and cancer and people we have loved who are not here any more because they smoked, the Voice has nothing to say. Have you noticed? Because I have and it is one of my defences against smoking again. When that urge gets almost unbearable I remember Pop; I handle his tobacco tin lovingly and understand why he isn't here, why he was missing in action so young, so stupidly, so pointlessly. I listen for what the Voice has to say and it is silent.

Smoking represents to me being grown up. When I was a kid I hated being a kid. I wanted to be grown up more than anything else. Smoking was my passport out of childhood; my ticket to the adult world. I suppose it could just as easily have been alcohol or thieving or sex. Alright, it was this last one also but this isn't so health risking or addictive (ha!). When I was fifteen I tried to get in to see the film Day Of The Triffids (an X certificate – you couldn't see it under sixteen). I pulled my collar up and stuck a fag in my mouth to look older, more grown up. The ruse didn't work. I was duly thrown out and quite right too – it really was a dreadful film, as I came to realise later when I did see it. But it was the fag which I thought gave me the aura of grown upness. Children don't smoke. Grown ups smoke. Therefore if I don't smoke I have reverted to childhood. Mind you at my age that might not be such a bad thing.

Order form

You can order any of our books via any of the contact routes on page 165, including on our website. Or fill out the order form below and fax it or post it to us.

We'll normally send your copy out by first class post within 24 hours (but please allow five days for delivery). We don't charge postage and packing within the UK. Please add £1 per book for postage outside the UK.

Title (Mr/Mrs/Miss/Ms/Dr/Lord etc)

Name

Address

Postcode

Daytime phone number

Email

No. of copies	Title	Price	Total £
	Postage and packing £1 per book (outside the UK only):		
	TOTAL:		

Please either send us a cheque made out to White Ladder Press Ltd or fill in the credit card details below.

Type of card ☐ Visa ☐ Mastercard ☐ Switch

Card number

Start date (if on card) _____ Expiry date _____ Issue no (Switch) _____

Name as shown on card

Signature

slides sideways, narrowly avoiding hitting one already parked. I realise it would be a terrible irony to survive a stroke and then get run over in the hospital car park, and so I head back inside, grateful for once that the temperature in the Gainsborough Wing is close to that of a greenhouse at Kew Gardens.

The ascent of the stairwell takes about four times longer than the descent, but I finally make it, bathed in sweat and incredibly pleased with myself. Going up and down those stairs at least once a day, sometimes twice, becomes my personal exercise regime. On the ground floor there is a little shop run by volunteer 'Friends of the Hospital' which sells sweets, snacks, fruit, flowers and newspapers to both patients and visitors. It gives me the perfect excuse to use those stairs: in the mornings to get a newspaper and then in the afternoon to buy some sweets for the kids when they visit (though I try and drop the hint that they are supposed to bring me gifts).

I don't tell anyone I'm doing this, and certainly no other Birch Ward patient is, but as I am no longer being offered physiotherapy, it is the only exercise I get.

Some days I get dressed for these excursions and even venture over into the main hospital where there is a bigger shop which also sells second hand books and I even find an ex-library edition of a William McIlvanney novel I had not heard of, which cheers me up no end. Returning to Birch Ward after one of these jaunts, I am mistaken for a visitor to the ward by a family of real visitors looking for a patient in a private room. I hadn't known there were private rooms, so I take them to the nurses' station where Bill, one of the senior male nurses, says they've been looking for me to take my blood pressure and would I mind getting back in my bed.

One morning the cheeky young nurse – Louisa (a short brunette with bags of attitude) – announces loudly:

"Come on, Mike. Let's do some drugs!"

Then, under her breath: "It's only aspirin, I'm afraid."

Nurse Bill explains that I will probably be taking a small daily dose of aspirin (75mg, sometimes known as 'half-aspirin' or, in America, 'baby aspirin') as well as other drugs for the rest of my life and they need to see if I can cope with 'self-medication'. This is nothing more than opening the bottle and taking a small tablet once a day, but I am watched like a hawk for the first few days to make sure I can manage, or, more likely, to make sure I don't forget.

REDUCING HIGH BLOOD PRESSURE

If your blood pressure is not too high, non-pharmacological treatments can be effective – which is a very fancy way of saying you don't always need to take drugs. These treatments revolve around diet and what is nowadays known as 'lifestyle'.

Family doctors are often criticised for failing to explain to patients how to change their lifestyle, but then very few patients want 'boring' advice about losing weight and stopping smoking as it involves giving up things they like. A far easier prescription would be a magic pill which does it all for you even though one does not, as yet, exist.

Reducing the body's sodium intake and increasing the potassium intake is important for blood pressure. This is a very fancy way of saying take less salt and eat more fruit.

Victims with high cholesterol levels have to be more careful and take advice on reducing their fat intake. Statins, the drugs given to lower cholesterol, have been proved to work better in conjunction with a diet.

Exercise is always mentioned as being good for hypertension, with even as little as a 30-minute brisk walk every day making a difference.

Relaxing – simply taking it easy – has no real effect, though some practitioners maintain that whilst Yoga won't actually lower high blood pressure, it is good for maintaining a steady level once it has come down.

Neither alcohol nor smoking have long-term effects on blood pressure directly, but smoking can clog up the arteries (which does have an effect) and of course can be linked to lung and heart disease. Alcohol actually gives some protection against heart disease, but doesn't help if you are trying to lose weight.

I begin to press the nurses for more information on what the future might hold for me, though it still doesn't occur to me to ask about my blood pressure, which is ritually being measured twice a day.

I'm told that the results of my CT or CAT scan are now known, though of course the consultant hasn't seen them because he's off sick.

The Computerised Tomography scan (or Computed Axial Tomography), has confirmed that I suffered a blood clot on the right side of the brain, which had affected the left side of my body. In technical terms, I learn that this was 'a right internal capsule infarct'.

No one is saying what might have caused it, but Nurse Bill says the smoking "can't have helped" and asks if anyone has said anything about giving up? I tell him not officially, though I haven't had a cigarette for eleven days, eight hours and 43 minutes – not that I was counting, of course. He suggests nicotine patches and later that day he brings me a supply, but I don't actually start to use them until after I am discharged.

Although I had smoked about 20 cigarettes a day for over 25 years, I had always associated smoking with concentration on a piece of work, not relaxation. I could quite happily watch a film or a play without a cigarette and often go an entire weekend without one, but back at work in the office, or sitting at home in front of a computer screen or the blank sheet of paper in a typewriter, I would automatically reach for my cigarettes and lighter. I always grabbed a cigarette when the phone rang, something which used to drive Alyson crazy. It is her threat to break my fingers if she finds me with a cigarette which will be far more effective than nicotine patches in the long run.

During the family's evening visit, I tell Aly about the CT scan and she agrees to email one of our American friends, Ray Daniloff. Ray is a professor of Audiology at the University of

*Texas, and teaches people to be speech therapists. Both person-
ally and professionally he has experience of heart problems
and strokes, and has been emailing for a diagnosis since it
happened.*

*I tell Aly to reply with the words "right side – clot, not bleed"
only, which she does and he responds with: "You have, my
friend, avoided a very bad bullet".*

Stop Smoking, Stay Cool

A dedicated smoker's guide to not smoking

RICHARD CRAZE

Any stroke sufferer who smokes will be strongly advised to give up. It's easy to say, but much harder to do. *Stop Smoking, Stay Cool* is Richard Craze's honest and funny account of giving up smoking after dedicating himself to tobacco for over 30 years. His journal holds the reader's hand through withdrawal symptoms, mood swings, coughs, mouth ulcers and all the other symptoms, including The Voice. He offers real help for those wanting to give up, and especially those who see smoking as cool (which is, frankly, most smokers) and don't want to sacrifice their personal image when they quit the fags.

If you'd like to order a copy of the book, it costs £7.99 and is available via any of the routes on page 166, or you can use the order form at the back of this book.

Stop Smoking, Stay Cool

DAY 20

As I approach the end of my first three weeks without tobacco I am questioning my identity as a 'not smoking at the moment thank you' sort of person. I mean, who is this new smelling of soap chap I have become? When I smoked I was a smoker; that was me. I smoked roll ups. I smelt of tobacco and tweed and damp corduroy. I was relaxed and chilled. I wore John Lennon glasses and read Stephen King and liked a nice cup of tea (mind you I am drinking upwards of twenty cups a day now; is that another addiction I shall have to address in time?) and walking my dogs across fields where I could lean on a farm gate and have a roll up and watch the clouds and internally philosophise about life and death and the universe and everything.

Now I am sharp with the children, cold and fresh, smelling of carbolic, afraid to sit still for too long in case I give in to this damn ridiculous voice in my head, unable to work or sleep, eating too much, a neurotic bundle of twitches and jerks. I mean, who am I now? Do I approve of who I have become? Am I the sort of person I wouldn't have shared a railway carriage with before? Have I become a New Man? I liked the old me, the smelly, slightly singed around the edges me. I have become...no, I can't say it...I have become...a non smoker. Arg! I can hear the Voice mocking me.

You see smoking is so attractive. Smoking is rebellious, young, carefree. It makes such a defiant statement about who you are. If you smoke you are signing up to wearing a leather jacket with the collar turned up, listening to rock and roll, staying up late, talking about life, the universe and everything, rebelling and behaving like a grown up. Now you are washed and ready for bed after your tea. You are a child again. You smell nice, but of nothing real or grown up or dangerous. You have gone from being James Dean to Wendy Craig in one swift stubbing out of a fag. You are a disappointment to me.

And to myself. I could almost weaken. This is such a persuasive argument. I could, almost. I do like the idea of smoking a pipe. I've always thought the smell of damp tweed and pipe tobacco a good thing.

My grandfather smoked roll ups. He had a silver tobacco tin with a sun burst engraved on it. How do I remember it so clearly? I have it by me as I write. My uncle gave it to me to remember Pop by. I used it for many years myself but it is now redundant. Pop died of emphysema/bronchitis/pneumonia, due to his smoking, at the age of sixty eight. I don't think a day goes by when I don't think of him and miss him. I didn't have a father so my grandfather was the nearest I got to a role model/father figure. Is this why I have smoked so long, so often, so much? I have to question it. To beat this Voice I have to know why I smoked.

My grandfather rolled roll ups gently, with time and care and, as a small boy, I would watch him fascinated, hypnotised, in rapture. I loved the smell of them, of him. It's easy now to remember the hawking cough which I blanked at the time, and the fact that it was smoking which killed him. It also killed my mother at the age of seventy. Did she smoke because her beloved dad did? Were we all trying to be like Pop? To be Pop? He was the kindest, funniest man ever. We all loved him.

Notice how the Voice goes quiet when the serious business of smoking comes up? When we talk of death and cancer and people we have loved who are not here any more because they smoked, the Voice has nothing to say. Have you noticed? Because I have and it is one of my defences against smoking again. When that urge gets almost unbearable I remember Pop; I handle his tobacco tin lovingly and understand why he isn't here, why he was missing in action so young, so stupidly, so pointlessly. I listen for what the Voice has to say and it is silent.

Smoking represents to me being grown up. When I was a kid I hated being a kid. I wanted to be grown up more than anything else. Smoking was my passport out of childhood; my ticket to the adult world. I suppose it could just as easily have been alcohol or thieving or sex. Alright, it was this last one also but this isn't so health risking or addictive (ha!). When I was fifteen I tried to get in to see the film Day Of The Triffids (an X certificate – you couldn't see it under sixteen). I pulled my collar up and stuck a fag in my mouth to look older, more grown up. The ruse didn't work. I was duly thrown out and quite right too – it really was a dreadful film, as I came to realise later when I did see it. But it was the fag which I thought gave me the aura of grown upness. Children don't smoke. Grown ups smoke. Therefore if I don't smoke I have reverted to childhood. Mind you at my age that might not be such a bad thing.